Multidisciplinary Management of Acute and Chronic Pancreatitis

Edited by Marco Massani and Tommaso Stecca

Published in London, United Kingdom

Multidisciplinary Management of Acute and Chronic Pancreatitis
http://dx.doi.org/10.5772/intechopen.101001
Edited by Marco Massani and Tommaso Stecca

Contributors
Christos Damaskos, Nikolaos Garmpis, Dimitrios Dimitroulis, Dionysios Prevezanos, Anna Garmpi, Gregory Kouraklis, Arda Yavuz, Agostino Paccagnella, Maria Lisa Marcon, Maria Sara Persano, Claudia Vigo, Elisa Paccagnella, Giovanni Morana, Alessandro Beleù, Francesca Nistri, Silvia Venturini, Michael Okello, Derick Kayondo, Mariana Chávez-Tostado, Karla Verónica Chávez-Tostado, Mario Alberto Ramírez-Herrera, Maria Luisa Mendoza-Magaña, Gabino Cervantes-Guevara, Alejandro González-Ojeda, Clotilde Fuentes-Orozco, Guillermo Alonso Cervantes-Cardona, Diana Mercedes Hernánez-Corona, Tonatiuh González-Heredia, Milton Omar Guzmán-Ornelas, Miriam Méndez-del Villar, María Fernanda Isadora Meraz-Corona, Enrique Cervantes-Pérez, Abraham Alberto Ramírez-Mendoza, Steffany Arandeni Ramírez-Mendoza, Tommaso Stecca, Marco Massani, Cristina Nistri, Bruno Pauletti, Adriana Di Giacomo, Flavio Colaut, Mariangela Ruperto, Ezio Caratozzolo, Luca Bonariol, Annapaola Dotto, Eleonora Pinese, Ilenia Barbuscio, Stefano Benvenuti

First published in London, United Kingdom, 2023 by IntechOpen
IntechOpen is the global imprint of INTECHOPEN LIMITED, registered in England and Wales, registration number: 11086078, 5 Princes Gate Court, London, SW7 2QJ, United Kingdom

British Library Cataloguing-in-Publication Data
A catalogue record for this book is available from the British Library

Additional hard and PDF copies can be obtained from orders@intechopen.com

Multidisciplinary Management of Acute and Chronic Pancreatitis
Edited by Marco Massani and Tommaso Stecca
p. cm.
Print ISBN 978-1-80356-158-5
Online ISBN 978-1-80356-159-2
eBook (PDF) ISBN 978-1-80356-160-8

For EU product safety concerns:
IN TECH d.o.o., Prolaz Marije Krucifikse Kozulić 3, 51000 Rijeka, Croatia,
info@intechopen.com or visit our website at intechopen.com.

Meet the editors

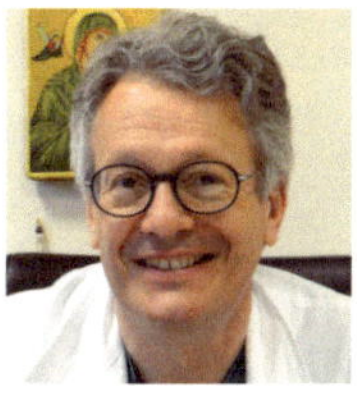

Dr. Marco Massani, MD, is a senior hepato-pancreato-biliary (HPB) surgeon. Since 2018, he has been the chief of the First Division of General Surgery, Referral Center for HPB Surgery, Ca' Foncello Treviso Regional Hospital, Italy. He received his surgical training at the University of Padova, Italy, and was educated both at home and abroad at the major HPB surgery centers of Memorial Sloan Kettering Cancer Center and Mount Sinai, both in New York. He is a member of multidisciplinary boards for colorectal and HPB diseases. He is a lecturer of liver surgery for the Italian School of Minimally Invasive Liver Surgery (I Go MILS) and for the Italian Society of Surgery. He is an active member of Italian and international surgical societies, including the International Hepato-Pancreato-Biliary Association (IHPBA), Società Italiana di Chirurgia (SIC), and Associazione Italiana di Chirurgia Epato-Bilio-Pancreatica (AICEP). He is the guest editor and invited reviewer *for Frontiers in Surgery* and the journal publisher *Multidisciplinary Digital Publishing Institute* (MDPI).

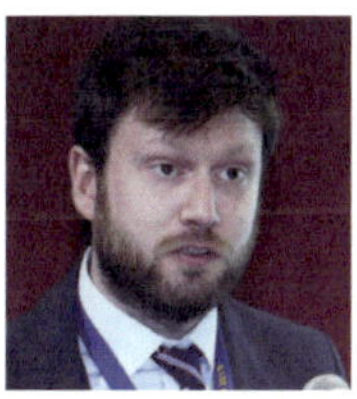

Dr. Tommaso Stecca is a general surgeon focused on hepato-pancreato-biliary (HPB) and colorectal disease. He graduated with an MD in 2012 and obtained a specialization in general surgery at the University of Padua, Italy, in 2018. He is an attending surgeon in the Department of Surgery, Treviso Regional Hospital, Italy, directed by Dr. Marco Massani. Between 2010 and 2014, Dr. Stecca also practiced in a research laboratory focused on the isolation and characterization of biliary epithelial cells and stromal cells from resected human cholangiocarcinoma. Dr. Stecca is the author of numerous scientific publications and a member of the Italian Surgical Association (SIC), the Italian Chapter, the European-African and the International Hepato-Pancreato-Biliary Association (AICEP, EA-HPBA, IHPBA), the Society for Surgery of the Alimentary Tract (SSAT), and the Italian Society of Colorectal Surgery (SICCR). He is a reviewer for *Frontiers in Surgery* and the journal publisher *Multidisciplinary Digital Publishing Institute* (MDPI).

Contents

Preface

Most patients suffering from acute pancreatitis will have a mild, self-limited, and uncomplicated course. However, local and systemic complications, ranging from mild to life-threatening, can occur. These include pancreatic and/or peripancreatic fluid collections, walled-off necrosis, infected pancreatic necrosis, and chronic disease. The accuracy of the predictors of severity actually employed and related therapeutic choices are still under debate, and clinical practice is often discordant with clinical practice guidelines. This book reviews the physiology and pathophysiology of pancreatic secretion, surgical and endoscopic management in acute and chronic settings, fluid resuscitation and anesthesiologic management, benefits and limitations of early enteral or parenteral nutritional interventions in patients with acute pancreatitis, nutritional recommendations in patients with chronic pancreatitis, and the radiologic features of acute and chronic disease.

The successful management of patients with pancreatitis requires a multidisciplinary team composed of gastroenterologists, surgeons, interventional radiologists, and specialists in critical care medicine and nutrition.

This book provides an overview of the multidisciplinary treatment of pancreatitis, both in its acute and chronic form.

Dr. Marco Massani
Department of Surgery,
Chief, First General Surgery Division,
Hepato-Pancreato-Biliary Regional Referral Centre,
Azienda ULSS2 Marca Trevigiana,
Ospedale Ca' Foncello, Treviso, Italy

Dr. Tommaso Stecca
Department of Surgery,
First General Surgery Division,
Hepato-Pancreato-Biliary Regional Referral Centre,
Azienda ULSS2 Marca Trevigiana,
Ospedale Ca' Foncello, Treviso, Italy

Section 1

Management

Chapter 1

Management of Acute and Chronic Pancreatitis

Tommaso Stecca, Cristina Nistri, Bruno Pauletti, Adriana Di Giacomo, Flavio Colaut, Mariangela Ruperto, Ezio Caratozzolo, Luca Bonariol and Marco Massani

Abstract

Pancreatitis is a major public health issue worldwide. There is geographical variation in the burden of acute and chronic pancreatitis (CP). Globally, the age-standardized prevalence rate increased from 1990 to 2017. Acute pancreatitis (AP) is now one of the most common reasons for hospitalization with a gastrointestinal condition. The essential requirements for the management of AP are accurate diagnosis, appropriate triage, high-quality supportive care, monitoring for and treatment of complications, and prevention of relapse. Clinicians should be aware of the time course and the best management of AP, identifying which patient will have a severe course allowing earlier triage to an intensive care unit and earlier initiation of effective therapy. CP is a pathologic fibroinflammatory syndrome of the pancreas in individuals with genetic, environmental, and other risk factors who develop persistent pathologic responses to parenchymal injury or stress. Diagnosing the underlying pathologic process early in the disease course and managing the syndrome to change the natural course of disease and minimize adverse disease effects are the managing paradigm. In this review, we consider recent changes in the management of acute and CP, as well as common misunderstandings and areas of ongoing controversy.

Keywords: acute pancreatitis, chronic pancreatitis, management, clinical phases, pathologic process

1. Introduction

Pancreatitis is a major public health issue worldwide. There is geographical variation in the burden of acute and chronic pancreatitis (CP). Globally, the age-standardized prevalence rate increased from 1990 to 2017. Acute pancreatitis (AP) is now one of the most common reasons for hospitalization with a gastrointestinal condition. The essential requirements for the management of AP are accurate diagnosis, appropriate triage, high-quality supportive care, monitoring for and treatment of complications, and prevention of relapse. Clinicians should be aware of the time course and the best management of AP, identifying which patient will have a severe course allowing earlier triage to an intensive care unit and earlier initiation of effective therapy. CP is a pathologic fibroinflammatory syndrome of the pancreas in individuals with genetic, environmental, and other risk factors who develop persistent pathologic responses to parenchymal injury or stress. Diagnosing the underlying pathologic process early in the disease course and managing the syndrome to change the natural course of disease and minimize adverse disease effects is the managing paradigm. In this review, we consider recent changes in the management of acute and CP, as well as common misunderstandings and areas of ongoing controversy.

Current concepts of the use of interventional methods in severe acute, necrotizing, and CP (indications and timing of interventions, strategies for intervention, endoscopic and percutaneous treatment) are discussed in the other chapters of this monograph on pancreatitis. We, therefore, consider it appropriate that they are illustrated in detail in the respective chapters.

2. Acute pancreatitis

AP is an acute inflammatory condition of the pancreas with histological acinar cells destruction. It has a wide spectrum of morphological and clinical manifestations and can result in local injury, systemic inflammatory response syndrome (SIRS) and organ failure [1, 2].

2.1 Epidemiology

AP is one of the most common gastrointestinal diseases requiring acute hospitalization [3]. Its incidence is rising worldwide and ranges from 5 to 30 cases per 100,000 [1] and despite improvements in the diagnosis, management and treatment, the overall mortality rate of AP remains around 2–5% [4, 5]. The average length of hospital stay for AP is 8 days, with economic burden to patients and the health care system all around the world [6].

2.2 Etiology

The most common causes of AP are gallstones (up to 40–70% of cases) and alcohol abuse (25–35%).

Migrating gallstones cause transient obstruction of the pancreatic duct leading to the blockage of pancreatic secretion and lysosomal dysfunction generating injury and inflammatory response. Alcohol abuse exerts its effects in a complex way that include direct toxicity and immunologic mechanisms: prolonged alcohol use (four to five drinks in a day over a period of more than 5 years) is required and the type of alcohol ingested does not affect the overall lifetime risk of alcohol-associated pancreatitis, that range from 2% to 5% in heavy drinkers ("Heavy" alcohol consumption is generally considered to be >50 g in a day).

In absence of gallstones or alcohol, other etiologies of AP (**Table 1**) must be ruled out.

The agent or condition causing AP is not always clear and sometimes there is only the evidence of factors known to be potential contributors of unexplained pancreatitis, such as smoke, obesity and diabetes. Accordingly, idiopathic AP has been defined as a condition in which the etiological cause is not detectable after an accurate anamnesis excluding any substance abuse, infections, metabolic disorders, genetic mutations and at least two second-level imaging techniques [endoscopic ultrasound and

Cause	Frequency	Notes
Gallstones	40%	Gallbladder stones or sludge
Alcohol	25–35%	Usually an acute flares on underlying chronic pancreatitis
Drugs	<5%	Most strongly associated: azathioprine, 6-mercaptopurine, dideoxyinosine, valproic acid, angiotensin-converting-enzyme inhibitors, mesalamine
Hypertriglyceridemia	1–5%	Triglyceride level > 10 mmol/l (>1000 mg/dl)
Hypercalcemia		Total serum calcium concentration > 2.60 mmol/l
Autoimmune causes	<1%	Autoimmune pancreatitis (AIP), type 1 or type 2
Genetic causes	Not known	Mutations and polymorphisms in different genes encoding cationic trypsinogen (PRSS1), serine protease inhibitor Kazal type 1 (SPINK1), cystic fibrosis transmembrane conductance regulator (CFTR), chymotrypsin C, calcium-sensing receptor
Endoscopic Retrograde CholangioPancreatography (ERCP)	5–10%*	
Trauma	<1%	Blunt or penetrating trauma
Infections	<1%	CMV, mumps, EBV
Tumors		Malignant tumor of ampulla, distal choledocus or pancreatic head**
Other causes of obstruction	Rare	Pancreas divisum, sphincter of Oddi dysfunction, any benign or malignant mass that obstructs the main pancreatic duct**
Other conditions, unknow	Common	Diabetes, obesity, smoking

**Among patients undergoing ERCP. **5–14% of patients with benign or malignant pancreatobiliary tumors present with AP.*

Table 1.
Causes of acute pancreatitis.

magnetic resonance imaging (MRI)] to exclude abnormality of pancreatic gland, pancreatic or biliary and gallbladder lithiasis.

Any mass that obstructs the main pancreatic duct can cause AP: 5–14% of patients with benign or malignant pancreatobiliary tumors present with this scenario and pancreatic tumor should be suspected in any patient older than 40 years with idiopathic pancreatitis, especially those with prolonged or recurrent course [4–6].

2.3 Clinical signs and symptoms

Patients with AP usually present with epigastric or left upper quadrant pain, usually described as persistent, severe and often radiating to the back, chest or flanks. The intensity of pain is not correlated to the severity of the disease. Patients experience pain relief when sitting forward or worsening when lying flat. Nausea and vomiting are also common, and sequestered fluid in the small bowel may lead to rapid and severe dehydration. Diaphragmatic irritation may cause hiccoughs. The presentation can also be dominated by shock with tachycardia, tachypnea, hypotension, anuria and mental status alteration. On the other hand, patients may be paucisymptomatic, with few physical signs. Abdominal examination reveals epigastric tenderness and guarding; abdominal distension with paralytic ileus. Later signs may include mottled skin or livedo reticularis and lace-like purplish discoloration of the skin. Abdominal periumbilical ecchymosis (Cullen's sign) and ecchymosis of the flank (Grey Turner's sign) result from the diffusion of fat necrosis and inflammation associated with retroperitoneal or intra-abdominal bleeding [5].

2.4 Diagnosis

The diagnosis of AP is made following the Revised Atlanta Criteria, a global consensus classification (generated in 1992 and revised in 2012) designed to standardize diagnosis, clinical assessment, evaluation, severity and complications of AP and to help the communication between clinicians.

Diagnosis of AP requires two of the following three features:

- *abdominal pain consistent with AP*;
- *serum lipase or amylase levels at least three times greater than the upper limit of normal range*;
- *characteristic findings of AP on imaging* [contrast-enhanced computed tomography (CT) and less commonly MRI or transabdominal ultrasonography].

According to these criteria, it is important to underline that when the diagnosis of AP is established by abdominal pain and by increased serum pancreatic enzyme activities (clinical and laboratory criteria), the radiological findings (imaging criteria) are not required for making the diagnosis [3, 7].

In the majority of patients, routine use of CT or MRI is unwarranted as the diagnosis of AP is apparent and most have a mild, uncomplicated course. CT or MRI imaging should be reserved for patients in whom the diagnosis is unclear or who fail to improve clinically within the first 48–72 hours after hospital admission [6].

Contrarily, transabdominal ultrasound should be performed on admission in all patients with AP, to define the underlying etiology and to identify the presence of gallstones that are the most common cause of AP [3, 6].

Moreover, it is important to record the time interval between onset, first observation and hospital admission. In fact, the onset of AP is defined as the time of beginning of abdominal pain and not the time of admission to the hospital [7].

In an episode of AP, the enzyme secreted by the pancreas (amylase, lipase, elastase and trypsin) are released from acinar cells of the pancreas into the bloodstream at the same time, due to increased permeability following inflammation.

Amylase is an enzyme synthesized mostly by pancreatic acinar cells and salivary glands and in negligible levels by adipose tissue, gonads, fallopian tubes, intestinal tract and skeletal muscle. Humans product one specific isoenzyme, α-amylase, with two major isoforms specific to pancreas and to salivary glands that help to identify different cases of hyperamylasemia. In case of AP, serum amylase rises rapidly within a few hours after the onset, with peaks at 3–6 hours, half-life of 10–12 hours, persistent elevation for 3–5 days and decrease to normal levels over the next three to 7 days.

Lipase is an enzyme that has a higher specificity because is mainly produced by acinar cells of the pancreas; nevertheless, high serum level can be determined also in patient with renal insufficiency, appendicitis, diabetic ketoacidosis, inflammatory bowel disease and intestinal obstruction. In AP, elevation of serum lipase arises within three to 6 hours with peaks at 24 hours following the onset of symptoms and persistent elevation up to 2 weeks, giving a larger diagnostic window in comparison to amylase.

Therefore, serum lipase appears to be more specific and remains elevated for a longer period than serum amylase after disease presentation. Moreover, lipase has a better degree of sensitivity and specificity in diagnosing AP, during both early and late phases of the disease (sensitivity of lipase and amylase tests ranges between 64–100% and 45–87%, respectively).

According to these evidences, current guidelines recommend the preference use of serum lipase for diagnosis of AP [2, 4, 6].

2.5 Classification

The most commonly used classification system for AP is the “2012 revision of the Atlanta Classification and definitions” based on international consensus [8].

This classification identifies two types (Interstitial edematous pancreatitis and necrotizing pancreatitis), three grades of severity (mild, moderately severe or severe) and two phases (early and late) of AP.

2.5.1 Types of acute pancreatitis

Two different types of AP have been characterized: Interstitial edematous pancreatitis and necrotizing pancreatitis.

Interstitial edematous pancreatitis is an acute inflammation of pancreatic parenchyma and peri-pancreatic tissues, but without recognizable tissue necrosis. Developed by the majority of patients (80–85%), it is characterized by diffuse (or occasionally localized) enlargement of the pancreas, due to inflammatory edema; the clinical symptoms usually resolve within the first week.

Necrotizing pancreatitis is, instead, the presence of inflammation associated with pancreatic parenchymal necrosis and/or peri-pancreatic necrosis. The natural history of necrotizing pancreatitis is variable and this scenario evolves over several days because necrosis can remain solid or liquefy, can remain sterile or become infected, persist or disappear over time. This explains why an early CT made for assessment of AP may underestimate the eventual extent of pancreatic and peri-pancreatic necrosis. Moreover, most evidence suggest no correlation between the extent of necrosis and the risk of infection and duration of symptoms and usually infected necrosis is rare during the first week. Developed by 15–20% of patients with AP, this type of evolution of AP has increased morbidity and mortality compared to patients with interstitial edematous pancreatitis [5, 7].

2.5.2 Severity of acute pancreatitis

A preliminary overview of complications of AP is mandatory, because the comprehension of these terminologies is central to definition and stratification of severity.

- **Local complications**: acute peri-pancreatic fluid collection, pancreatic pseudocyst, acute necrotic collection (sterile or infected), walled of necrosis (sterile or infected), gastric outlet dysfunction, splenic and portal vein thrombosis, ischemic colitis, colonic necrosis, enteric fistulas, hemorrhages.

- **Systemic complications**: exacerbation of preexisting comorbidities, such as chronic obstructive pulmonary disease, coronary artery disease or chronic liver disease.

- **Organ failure** is defined using the modified Marshall scoring system, that has the advantage of being simple, universally applicable, objective and easily repeatable daily. In AP three organ systems have to be assessed: respiratory, cardiovascular and renal. Respiratory failure is defined with a PaO_2/FiO_2 ratio <300, cardiovascular failure with a systolic blood pressure <90 mmHg non responsive to fluid administration and renal failure with a serum creatinine level ≥1.9 mg/dl (**Table 2**) [7, 9]. If organ failure affects more than one organ system, it is termed multiple organ failure (MOF).

- **Transient organ failure** is defined as organ failure existing for less than 48 hours, while **persistent organ failure** is organ failure persisting for more than 48 hours [7].

There are three degrees of severity of AP:

- **Mild AP**: absence of organ failure and absence of local or systemic complications

- **Moderately severe AP**: presence of transient organ failure (<48 hours) and/or presence of local or systemic complications (in absence of persistent organ failure)

- **Severe AP**: presence of persistent organ failure (>48 hours), that can involve single or multiple organs [7].

Usually, mild AP account for 80–85% of cases, while severe AP is reported in 15–30% of patients [6].

2.5.3 Phases of acute pancreatitis

AP is a dynamic disease with variable scenarios of evolution, but it has two overlapping phases that need to be considered separately to better understand the progression and consequences of this disease.

Organ system	**Parameter**	**Score**				
		0	**1**	**2**	**3**	**4**
Respiratory	PaO_2/FiO_2	>400	301–400	201–300	101–200	≤101
Cardiovascular	Systolic blood pressure (mmHg)	>90	<90, fluid responsive	<90, fluid unresponsive	<90, pH < 7.3	<90, pH < 7.2
Renal	Serum Creatinine (mg/dl)	<1.4	1.4–1.8	1.9–3.6	3.6–4.9	>4.9

Table 2.
Modified Marshall scoring system for definition of organ failure in acute pancreatitis. A score of two or more in any system defines the presence of organ failure.

Heart rate	>90 beats/minute
Core temperature	<36°C or >38°C
White blood cells count	<4000 cells/mm or >12000 cells/mm^3
Respiratory rate	>20 breaths/minute
$PaCO_2$	<32 mmHg

Table 3.
SIRS diagnostic criteria. The presence of two or more criteria defines the presence of SIRS.

The **early phase** usually takes place in the first and second weeks of the disease. It is characterized by the host response to local pancreatic injury and inflammation, with activation of the cytokine cascades that can lead to SIRS (**Table 3**).

In this phase the scenario of AP is still evolving and local complications may be recognized but they are mutable and inaccurate to determine the grade of severity. Furthermore, the morphologic changes due to local complications are not correlated to the extension of organ damage and the severity of organ failure [7].

Instead, the presence of SIRS and his persistence over time are known to be correlated to an increased risk of developing organ failure, are associated to high mortality and are established as early indicator of the likely severity of AP [2, 10, 11]. Persistent SIRS (>48 hours) is associated with a mortality rate of 25% compared with 8% of transient SIRS [3].

Consequently, the determinant of severity in the early phase of AP is the presence and duration of organ failure, that is assessed thorough clinical criteria [7] (see Section 2.6.1 Initial Assessment, **Table 4**) and appears to be related to the development and persistence of SIRS [6].

In this phase, death occurs as a result of the development, the persistence and the progressive nature of organ dysfunction; the reversal of early organ failure has been shown to be important in preventing morbidity and mortality in patient with AP.

Patient characteristic	Age > 55 years	
	Obesity (BMI > 30 kg/m^2)	
	Altered mental status	
	Comorbid disease	
Presence of SIRS	(see **Table 3**)	
Laboratory findings	BUN > 20 mg/dl or rising	*Signs of hypovolemia*
	HCT > 44% or rising	
	Elevated creatinine	
Radiology findings	Pleural effusion	
	Pulmonary infiltrates	
	Multiple or extensive extra pancreatic collections	

BMI, body mass index; BUN, blood urea nitrogen; HCT, hematocrit.

Table 4.
Intrinsic patient-related risk factors for the development of severe disease.

Therefore, if SIRS is identified in this phase of the disease, patients must be treated according to the treatment of a severe AP [6].

The **late phase** usually develops after the second week of the disease and can extent from weeks to months; it is delineated by the persistence of systemic signs of inflammation or by the presence of local complications. Consequently, this scenario develops only in patients with moderately severe or severe AP.

In this phase the disease is still evolving and local complications need to be assessed and characterized with radiological imaging because they may need a specific management. Therefore, although the main determinant of severity in this phase is the persistence of organ failure, the need of radiological definition of local complications requires both clinical and morphological criteria [7].

In the natural history of AP, half of all deaths occur in the first 2 weeks and are mainly due to failure of multiple organ systems while the other half occur after 2 weeks and are mainly due to pancreatic and extrapancreatic infections [5].

2.5.4 Prediction of severity

The three severity degrees of AP have distinct characterizations that have direct implications for clinical management and are associated with different outcome and mortality:

- **Mild AP**: self-limited disease that occurs in approximately 80–85% of patients [5]. By 48 hours after the admission, these patients typically would have substantially improved [6]. Radiological imaging is routinely not mandatory and discharge generally occurs during the early phase. Mortality is rare (<2%) [5, 7].

- **Moderately severe AP**: usually radiological imaging is required to assess the presence and extent of local complications, that may resolve without the need of intervention but that may request prolonged specialist support and care. Mortality is low (<5%) [5, 7].

- **Severe AP**: specific and aggressive treatment and specialist support and care are needed. Mortality is high, ranging from 36% to 50%, and reflects the presence and persistence of SIRS and the development of single or MOF [7, 11].

Persistent SIRS (more than 48 hours) is related to a mortality rate of 25.4% and persistent MOF is associated with a mortality reported to be as great as 42% [10]. Infection of the pancreatic and peripancreatic necrosis occurs in about 20–40% of patients and is associated with worsening organ dysfunctions [2].

Therefore, there are important reasons to define and stratify the severity of AP: the correlation between grade of severity and outcome and mortality, the need to identify patients with potentially severe AP that require aggressive early treatment, the need to identify patients that need transfer from a secondary care center to a specialist one or to intensive care unit, the need to stratify patients into subgroups based on the presence of organ failure and local or system complications to enable patient-tailored treatment that may require a variety of interventions.

Consistently with the definitions of the degrees of severity, the real severity of AP cannot be assessed on admission to the hospital or on first observation because it is not known whether the patient will have transient or persistent organ failure.

Moreover, the evolutions and changes of morphological features of local and systemic complications over time ensure that it is generally not necessary to perform radiological imaging during the first week of admission. When necessary, a CT scan performed 5–7 day after the admission is more reliable in establishing the presence and extent of local complications.

For all these reasons, the dynamic and evolving scenario that characterizes AP need to be reassessed on a daily bases in the early phase of the disease and convenient time points to re-evaluate the patients are usually 24 hours, 48 hours and 7 days after admission to the hospital [7].

Different predictors of severity of AP have been developed over time to improve clinical judgment, including single serum markers and scoring systems incorporating clinical, radiological and laboratory findings. The features of the best predictive criteria are: simplicity, universal applicability across international centers, ability to stratify disease severity easily and objectively, possibility for use at presentation and daily repetition.

Serum lipase or amylase levels are central to diagnosis of AP, but their degree on bloodstream and their decrease have no prognostic value [5, 7].

Many authors consider an acute-phase reactant, the **C-reactive protein** (CRP), as the "gold standard" for disease severity assessment. An elevated CRP concentration of greater than 150 mg/l indicates that AP will have a complicated course with a sensitivity of 85% in the first 72 hours after the onset of symptoms. The major drawback of CRP is that peak levels are reached only after 48–72 hours from the onset of symptoms and therefore is a predictor of severity that takes 72 hours to become accurate. Furthermore, CRP is not disease-specific and can be elevated in other inflammatory conditions [2, 12].

Procalcitonin (PCT) is another acute-phase protein considered as a valuable marker for the detection of severe pancreatitis, with a cut-off value of 0.5 ng/ml. An increased PCT concentration in AP should be observed since the onset of the disease and therefore it is useful in the early prediction of severe AP; nevertheless, some authors suggest that it is more beneficial to measure the PCT level within 24–36 hours from the occurrence of symptoms [13, 14]. A PCT value of 3.8 ng/ml or higher within 96 hours after the onset of symptoms indicated a pancreatic necrosis with a sensitivity and specificity of 93% and 79%. Moreover, an elevated PCT predicts infected necrosis in patients with confirmed pancreatic necrosis and has the ability to indicate a status of bacterial infection [2, 12–14].

Several scoring systems have been developed over time: Ranson score (1974) [15], Glasgow-Imrie score (1978) [16], Acute Physiology and Chronic Health Evaluation II (APACHE-II) (1983) [17], APACHE combined with scoring for obesity (APACHE-O), Simplified Acute Physiology Score (SAPS II) (1984) [18], CT Severity Index (CTSI) (1990) [19, 20], Bedside Index for Severity in Acute Pancreatitis (BISAP) (2008) [21], Harmless Acute Pancreatitis Score (HAPS) (2009) [22], Sequential Organ Failure Assessment (SOFA) (2013) [23], Japanese Severity Score (JPN) (2013 revision) [24].

Ranson score is moderately accurate in stratifying patients in terms of severity but required full 48 hours to be completed, with eleven criteria to be valuated (in additions, some data are not routinely ordered during hospitalization) [15, 25]. **APACHE-II** is very complex: it evaluates the chronic health score and 12 physiologic measurement, is not designed for day to day evaluation and is not specific for AP [2, 17, 25]. **CTSI** is based on local complications showed on CT scan findings and has the drawback of not reflecting the systemic inflammatory response [19, 20, 25]. **BISAP** is one of the most accurate, is very simple (only five criteria), applicable in every day clinical practice and easily applied in the early phases [2, 21, 25].

The International Association of Pancreatology (IAP) and the American Pancreatic Association (APA) evidence-based guidelines for the management of AP, advised the use of **SIRS** to predict severe acute pancreatitis (SAP) on admission and at 48 hours. SIRS can be diagnosed on the basis of four routine clinical measurement (**Table 3**) and persistent SIRS (>48 hours) is associated with MOF and mortality (25% compared with 8% of transient SIRS). Arguments to recommend SIRS over the other predictive scoring systems are widespread familiarity, simplicity and the possibility for repetitive measurements; none of the other scoring systems are considered clearly superior or inferior to (persistent) SIRS [3].

Evidence on the predictive performance of all these scoring systems is variable and their sensitivity and specificity for predicting severe AP range between 55% and 90%, depending on the cut-off value and the timing of scoring. Limitations of these scoring systems have been either the inability to obtain a complete score until at least 48 hours into the illness (missing a potentially valuable early therapeutic window) or the complexity of the scoring system itself [2, 12].

For all these reasons, there are no "gold standard" prognostic scores for predicting severe AP [2]. They are still useful to prove or exclude severe disease but they cannot replace ongoing evaluation by an experienced clinician and a good clinical judgment.

2.6 Management

2.6.1 Initial assessment

Severity score systems are complex, cumbersome and typically require 48 hours to become accurate.

In absence of any available test to determine severity, clinicians need to be aware of clinical finding associated with a severe course. These includes patient's age, comorbid health problems, body mass index, presence of SIRS, signs of hypovolemia (such as elevated blood urea nitrogen (BUN) or elevated hematocrit) and presence of pleural effusion (**Table 4**). These intrinsic patient-related risk factors for the development of severe disease should be used for initial risk assessment and to consequentially provide adequate initial management to patients presenting with AP [6].

2.6.2 Initial management

An adequate initial management should be provided to all patients presenting with AP and patients with organ failure and/or SIRS should be admitted to an intensive care unit whenever possible.

Initial management includes fluid resuscitation with early aggressive hydration, pain management and adequate nutrition. Routine use of prophylactic antibiotics in patients with severe AP and/or sterile necrosis is not recommended.

Early aggressive fluid administration, defined as 250–500 ml/hour of isotonic crystalloid solution, is an effective intervention that is most beneficial during the first 12–24 hours and should be provided to all patients (unless cardiovascular, renal or other related comorbidities preclude it, as the main risk is fluid overload). It amounts to a total infusion of 2500–4000 ml within the first 24 hours and it seems to be sufficient to reach the resuscitation goals within these first hours [2, 3, 5, 6]. Fluid requirement should be reassessed at frequent intervals within 6 hours of admission and for the next 24–48 hours [6]. The response to fluid resuscitation should be based on clinical monitoring of fluid status (heart rate < 120 beats/minute, mean arterial pressure between 65 and 85 mmHg, urinary output >0.5–1 ml/kg/hour) [3, 5] and on biochemical targets (such as decreasing BUN and hematocrit and maintaining normal creatinine) [5, 6].

Pain is the cardinal symptom of AP and its relief is a clinical priority. All patients must receive analgesia and there is no evidence about any restriction in pain medications: the best recommendations is to adhere to the most current acute pain management guidelines, in a multimodal approach including non-steroidal anti-inflammation drugs (NSAID), opioids, epidural analgesia and patient-controlled analgesia (PCA) [2].

In patients with mild AP there is no need for complete resolution of pain or normalization of pancreatic enzyme levels before oral **feeding** is started. A low-fat soft or solid diet is safe and can be started soon after admission in the absence of nausea, vomiting, severe abdominal pain and ileus [5, 6]. Need for nutritional support may be predicted in severe AP or over day 5 from admission if the symptoms continue to be severe or there is inability to oral feedings [5]. When artificial feeding is required, enteral nutrition should be the preferred treatment and it is recommended to prevent infectious complications. Nasogastric or nasoduodenal feeding are clinically equivalent. Total parenteral nutrition should be avoided and reserved for the cases in which the enteral route is not available, not tolerated or nutritional goals are not met [2, 6].

Infectious complications (both pancreatic and extrapancreatic) are a major cause of morbidity and mortality in patients with AP. Furthermore, patients with infected pancreatic necrosis have a higher mortality rate when compared with patients with sterile necrosis.

Although it was previously believed that preventing the development of infected necrosis was important, different trials have shown no benefit of prophylaxis with antibiotic therapy [5]. Now is established that the role of antibiotics is to treat confirmed infected necrosis instead of prevent infectious complications in patients with sterile necrosis. Antibiotics known to penetrate pancreatic necrosis are carbapenems (such as imipenem), quinolones, fluoroquinolones, clindamycin, piperacillin and metronidazole and their administration may be useful in delaying or avoiding intervention.

Consequently, routine use of prophylactic antibiotics in patients with any type of AP is not recommended unless infection is suspected or confirmed. Furthermore, routine use of antifungal agents, along with antibiotics, is not recommended. Nevertheless, antibiotics should be given for extrapancreatic infections such as cholangitis, catheter-acquired infections, bacteremia, urinary tract infections and pneumonia [2, 3, 6, 26].

There is no current available **pharmacologic therapy** to mitigate AP and current treatment is largely supportive. Considering that pancreatic injury is mediated by autodigestive enzymes, anti-secretory agents such as glucagon and somatostatin have been tested as potential therapies with limited results. Use of protease inhibitors agents (such as gabexate mesilate) have been studied with the aim of blocking intrapancreatic activation of digestive enzymes but several trials showed conflicting results on clinical benefit. Also administration of indomethacin and steroid therapy have been assessed in clinical trials but their role remains to be determined [27]. A recent Cochrane review about pharmacological intervention for AP stated that there was no evidence of difference in short-term mortality between the groups in any of the comparisons. Despite this evidence, the authors underlined that interventions with at least two clinical benefits were: octreotide (somatostatin analog), which was associated with fewer serious adverse events and a lower proportion of people with organ failure; and gabexate mesilate, which was associated with fewer adverse events and a lower proportion of people requiring an additional invasive intervention compared to inactive intervention [28].

2.6.3 Patient-tailored management (of late phase of acute pancreatitis)

Whether AP progresses to the late phase of the disease, patients may require a variety of interventions that go beyond the initial management. Patient-tailored management may include ERCP, endoscopic ultrasonography (EUS), endoscopic and/or radiological drainage or surgical intervention for treatment of local complications and referral for cholecystectomy to prevent recurrent attacks and potential biliary sepsis [6].

ERCP is indicated in patients with biliary pancreatitis with common bile duct obstruction and/or cholangitis [3, 5].

Asymptomatic acute peripancreatic fluid collections and asymptomatic pseudocysts do not require therapy. The development of infection in the necrotic collection is the main indicator for therapy and treatment should be delayed preferably for more than 4 weeks [3, 5, 6]. Clinical and imaging signs are accurate and routine percutaneous fine needle aspiration and culture is not required [3, 5].

The optimal intervention strategy is always a step-up approach: initial broad-spectrum antibiotics administration, subsequent percutaneous radiological interventions followed, if needed, by endoscopic transmural drainage or endoscopic debridement and eventually by surgical approach [3, 5, 6]. Minimally invasive operative methods of necrosectomy and minimally invasive surgical approaches are always preferred to open necrosectomy [6]. The optimal strategy must be individualized for every patient and should be discussed by a multidisciplinary group of experts.

To prevent recurrence of AP, cholecystectomy should be performed before discharge in patient with mild gallstone AP. In this subgroup of patients, cholecystectomy performed 25–30 days after discharge has a higher rate of complications as compared with cholecystectomy performed during the initial hospitalization and a delay of cholecystectomy for more than a few weeks is associated with a high risk of relapse (up to 30%) of AP. Instead, in patient with necrotizing biliary AP, cholecystectomy should be delayed until active inflammation and fluid collections resolve or stabilize [3, 6]. In AP without biliary etiology, other protective measures to prevent relapses are mandatory such as smoking cessation, abstinence of alcohol intake, withdraw of implicated medications and tight control of hyperlipidemia.

2.7 Long-term consequences

Approximately 20–30% of patients develop pancreatic exocrine and endocrine dysfunction after AP and 30–50% of those patients will evolve in CP. Risk factors for these long-term consequences are the etiology, the severity and the degree of pancreatic necrosis of the initial attack of AP [5].

3. Chronic pancreatitis

CP is a clinical entity resulting from progressive inflammation and irreversible fibrosis of the pancreas due to cumulative damage to the pancreas over time.

It is a disease with various manifestations that can severely affect quality of life, while its long-term complications such as exocrine pancreatic insufficiency (EPI), diabetes mellitus, and risk of pancreatic cancer can become life-threatening. Diagnosis of CP can be challenging because, despite recent advances in imaging technology, radiologic findings are not apparent until late stages of the disease.

Only dynamic observation of patients with controlled follow-up allows us to classify pancreatitis and better define the disease by assigning definitive labels supported by biochemical and radiological sources that are well characterized by the various classification systems available. The clinician should recognize pancreatitis at an early stage but avoid making a "definitive" classification immediately.

3.1 Definition

In the last decade, advances in clinical and translational sciences have redefined our understanding of CP, thus changing the definition, the diagnosis and the management of the disease.

The traditional clinopathologic-based definition described CP as a *"a continuing inflammatory disease of the pancreas, characterized by irreversible morphological change, and typically causing pain and/or permanent loss of function"*. Such a diagnostic assessment resulted in a delay between symptom onset and diagnosis, failing to identify the underlying etiology, without predicting the clinical course or guide preventative treatments, being limited to symptomatic or supportive care and replacement of lost gland function [29].

In 2016, a new Mechanistic Definition of CP was published and adopted worldwide. This definition affirmed the characteristics of end-stage disease (**Table 5**) and addressed the disease mechanism as *"a pathologic fibroinflammatory syndrome of the pancreas in individuals with genetic, environmental, and/or other risk factors who develop persistent pathologic responses to parenchymal injury or stress"*. The new paradigm is to focus on diagnosing the mechanistic disorder underlying the pathogenic process early in the disease course and managing the syndrome to change the natural course and to minimize adverse disease effects. Within this framework it is important to recognize the difference between pancreatic dysfunction, pancreatitis-related disorders, and pancreatic disease [30, 31].

Pancreatic atrophy
Fibrosis
Pain syndromes
Duct distortion and strictures
Calcifications
Pancreatic exocrine dysfunction
Pancreatic endocrine dysfunction
Dysplasia

Table 5.
Characteristics of end-stage chronic pancreatitis.

3.2 Epidemiology

The epidemiology of CP is poor compared with other illnesses. There are few studies that look at the population distribution of CP, and it is important to note that these data are not available from large parts of the world. This is likely related to the difficulties in conducting such studies due to the low prevalence of the disease, the establishment of an accurate diagnosis, and the focus of previous studies on describing the clinical profile and natural history of the disease. Over the past two decades, there has been an interest in documenting the distribution of pancreatic disease in the population. Incidence of CP is currently estimated between 4.4 and 14 per 100,000 people, with a prevalence of 36.9–52.4 per 100,000 persons, and a male predominance by a factor of 1.5–4.6 [32, 33]

In 2016, a systematic review by Xiao et al. [34], that included only high-quality studies conducted on general populations, demonstrated a global pooled incidence of CP of 10 cases per 100,000 general population per year.

A recent 25-year population-based Danish study by Olesen et al. evaluated the incidence and the prevalence of CP between 1994 and 2018. The mean incidence rate was 12.6 per 100,000 person years for the total population; 8.6 vs. 16.7 per 100,000 person years in women and men, respectively. The Authors demonstrated that over a 25-year observation period the prevalence of CP was increasing in the Danish population (from 126.6 in 1996 to 153.9 in 2016), while the incidence remained stable; the mean age at CP diagnosis increased by almost a decade (52.1–60.0 years) [35].

3.3 Etiology

3.3.1 Risk factors

The most common risk factor for CP is alcohol abuse [36, 37]. In 1995, a study from Levy et al. demonstrated a logarithmic relationship between the relative risk of developing CP and the quantity of consumed alcohol, although the type of alcohol consumed is irrelevant [38]. There is not a threshold value, but a minimum of 80 g alcohol per day for a period of at least 6 years is considered to be a risk factor for the development of CP. An average of 18 ± 11 years elapses between the start of excessive alcohol consumption and the development of pancreatitis [39, 40].

Smoking is an independent risk factor. It accelerates the progression of CP, even with alcohol abstinence. It leads to pancreatic pain exacerbations and to calcifications. All patients should be advised to quit smoking [41–43]. In 2009, Yadav et al. published the results of the North American Pancreatitis Study 2 that prospectively enrolled 540 patients with CP. A dose-dependent association between smoking and CP was demonstrated; and patients without an history of alcohol but with 21–35 pack years have an increased risk of CP with a 3.26 odds ratio [44].

Primary hyperparathyroidism (pHPT) can lead to CP, with or without calcifications. 1% of patients with CP suffers from pHPT, conversely 12% of patients with pHPT also have pancreatitis, thus leading to a 28-fold increased risk of developing pancreatitis in this cohort of patients [45, 46].

Whether the anatomic anomaly pancreas divisum (the most common congenital malformation of the pancreas) is a risk factor for the development of CP is still a matter of debate. The S3-consensus conference on CP have reached an agreement on the following statement: "the presence of pancreas divisum without any further risk factors tend not to lead to chronic pancreatitis" [47].

Several genes have been associated with the diagnosis of CP. Genetic testing aim is to provide early information about the etiology of disease-related disorders that are contributing to the pathogenic process, to assist in decision making, and to help prevent the development of irreversible CP [48].

The most important genetic risk factors are variants in cationic trypsinogen (PRSS1), SPINK1 and carboxypeptidase A1 (CPA1). Further genetic susceptibility genes are CFTR, chymotrypsinogen C (CTRC) and carboxyesterlipase (CEL) [49–54].

Trypsinogen is a key molecule in the pathogenesis of pancreatitis, up to 66% of patients with hereditary pancreatitis have a mutation of the PRSS1 gene. Such mutations lead to CP with a penetrance of up to 80% and an autosomal dominant inheritance pattern [55–58].

Mutations of the SPINK1 gene predispose to idiopathic CP, occurring in as many as 30% of patients, however only in 1–2% of the general population. The N34S mutation in the gene encoding SPINK1 bears an odds ratio of 11.0 in developing CP.

Cystic fibrosis is an autosomal recessive disease with an estimated incidence of 1:2500. The first description of an association between CFTR variants and CP was published in 1998 [59]. The association between gene mutations and CP has an odds ratio of around 3–5 [55, 60]. CP patients carrying CFTR variants harbor at least one mild variant allele giving them residual CFTR function. Pancreas involvement may vary from a complete loss of exocrine and endocrine function to almost normal function. Molecular changes in the CFTR gene are associated to up to 30% of patients with idiopathic pancreatitis.

Patients with a CTRC mutation have an increased risk of developing CP. The first report dates back to 2008 [52]. Such mutations occur in 3.3% of patients with idiopathic pancreatitis.

In addition to those etiologic factors, autoimmune pancreatitis has been recently characterized. First reported in 1961 by Sarles [61], Yoshida first postulated this clinical entity in 1995 [62]. This is a systemic fibroinflammatory disease in which the pancreas is one of the affected organs. Men are affected twice than women. Clinical symptoms include abdominal pain, jaundice and recurrent episodes of pancreatitis. Radiological findings include "sausage-shaped pancreas" and diffuse or segmental Wirsung stenosis, often without prestenotic dilation. Serum levels of immunoglobulin (Ig) G and IgG4 have been found increased in the Asian patients, but only in 50% of European ones. Diagnosis is reached according to the HiSORT criteria (**Table 6**) [63] which include histology, serology, other organ involvement and response to steroid therapy [64–66].

3.3.2 Classification models

Distinct classification systems have been developed but, so far, no globally accepted classification system has been established. Classification systems currently in use are: Manchester classification; ABC classification; M-ANNHEIM; TIGAR-O; and Rosemont classification. Only the Toxic/metabolic, Idiopathic, Genetic, Autoimmune, Recurrent acute pancreatitis, and Obstructive (TIGAR-O) and the pancreatitis with Multiple risk factors-Alcohol consumption, Nicotine consumption, Nutritional factors, Hereditary factors, Efferent duct factors, Immunological factors, Miscellaneous and rare metabolic factors (M-ANNHEIM) classification systems take the etiology of CP into account.

The M-ANNHEIM system is a multirisk factor classification system. It adds information on disease activity and stage, evaluating the role of various risk factors on the

Category	Criteria
Histology	One of the following: 1. Periductal lymphoplasmacytic infiltrate with obliterative phlebitis and storiform fibrosis (LPSP) 2. Lymphoplasmacytic infiltrate with storiform fibrosis showing abundant IgG4 positive cells (≥10 cells/HPF)
Imaging CT/MRI	Typical: diffusely enlarged gland with diffuse rim enhancement, diffusely irregular attenuated pancreatic duct Other: focal pancreatic mass or enlargement; focal pancreatic duct stricture; pancreatic duct stricture, pancreatic atrophy; pancreatic calcification or pancreatitis
Serology	Elevated serum IgG4 level (>135 mg/dl)
Other organ involvement	Hilar/intrahepatic biliary strictures, persistent distal biliary strictures, parotid or lacrimal gland involvement, mediastinal lymphadenopathy or retroperitoneal fibrosis
Response to steroid therapy	Resolution/marked improvement of pancreatic/extrapancreatic manifestation with steroid therapy

LPSP, lymphoplasmacytic sclerosing pancreatitis; CT, computed tomography; MRI, magnetic resonance imaging; IgG4, immunoglobulin G4; HPF, high powered field.

Table 6.
The Mayo clinic HiSORT criteria for the diagnosis of AIP.

course of CP [67]. Relying upon traditional clinicopathologic criteria, and resulting in a score between 0–25, it provides diagnostic criteria for etiology, clinical and diagnostic stage (**Table 7**).

The TIGAR-O classification system comprises six etiologic groups: toxic-metabolic, idiopathic, genetic, autoimmune, recurrent AP, and obstructive groups. It

Clinical feature	Points
Patient report of pain	
No pain without therapy	0
Recurrent acute pancreatitis (RAP)	1
No pain with therapy	2
Intermittent pain	3
Continuous pain	4
Pain control	
No medication	0
Use of nonopioid drugs or use of mild opioids (WHO step 1 or 2)	1
Use of potent opioids (WHO step 3) or endoscopic intervention	2
Surgical intervention	
Pancreatic surgical intervention for any reason	4
Exocrine insufficiency	
Absence of exocrine insufficiency	0
Presence of mild, moderate, or unproven exocrine insufficiency not requiring enzyme supplementation (including patient reports of intermittent diarrhea)	1
Presence of proven exocrine insufficiency (according to exocrine function tests) or presence of marked exocrine insufficiency defined as steatorrhea (>7 g fat/24 hour), normalized or markedly reduced by enzyme supplementation	2

Clinical feature	Points
Endocrine insufficiency	
Absence of diabetes mellitus	0
Presence of diabetes mellitus	4
Morphologic status on pancreatic imaging (according to Cambridge classification)	
Normal	0
Equivocal	1
Mild	2
Moderate	3
Marked	4
Severe organ complications	
Absence of complications	0
Presence of possibly reversible complications	2
Presence of irreversible complications	4

Table 7.
The M-ANNHEIM scoring system for the grading of clinical features of chronic pancreatitis.

has been validated in multiple international studies, and in 2019 it was revised to include new insights from the past 20 years. It is designed as a hierarchical checklist to quickly document and track specific factors that may contribute to progressive pancreatic disease (**Table 8**) [68].

Toxic-metabolic
Alcohol-related (susceptibility and/or progression) 3–4 drinks/day 5 or more drinks/day Smoking (if yes, record pack-years) Non-smoker (<100 cigarettes in lifetime) Past smoker Current smoker Other, NOS Hypercalcemia (total calcium levels >12.0 mg/dl or 3 mmol/l) Hypertriglyceridemia Hypertriglyceridemic risk (fasting > 300 mg/dl; non-fasting > 500 mg/dl) Hypertriglyceridemic acute pancreatitis, history of (>500 mg/dl in first 72 hours) Medications (name) Toxins, other Chronic kidney disease (CKD)—(CKD Stage 5: end-stage renal disease, ESRD) Other, NOS Metabolic, other Diabetes Mellitus (with the date of diagnosis if available) Other, NOS
Idiopathic
Early onset (<35 years of age) Late onset (>35 years of age)
Genetic
Suspected; no or limited genotyping available Autosomal dominant (Mendelian inheritance—single gene syndrome) PRSS1mutations (hereditary pancreatitis) Autosomal recessive (Mendelian inheritance—single gene syndrome)

CFTR, 2 severe variants in *trans* (cystic fibrosis) CFTR, <2 severe variants in *trans* (CFTR-RD) SPINK1,2 pathogenic variants in *trans* (SPINK1-associated familial pancreatitis) Complex genetics (non-Mendelian, complex genotypes ± environment) Modifier genes (list pathogenic genetic variants) PRSS1-PRSS1 locus CLDN2 locus Others Hypertriglyceridemia (list pathogenic genetic variants) Other, NOS
AIP/steroid responsive pancreatitis
AIP Type 1—IgG4-related disease AIP Type 2
RAP and SAP
Acute pancreatitis (single episode, including date of event if available) AP etiology—extra-pancreatic (excluding alcoholic, HTG, hypercalcemia, genetic) Biliary pancreatitis Post-ERCP Traumatic Undetermined or NOS RAP (number of episodes, frequency, and dates of events if available)
Obstructive
Pancreas divisum Ampullary stenosis Main duct pancreatic stones Widespread pancreatic calcifications Main pancreatic duct strictures Localized mass causing duct obstruction

Table 8.
The TIGAR-O Version 2.0 risk/etiology classification, short form.

3.4 Diagnosis

The diagnosis is made using a combination of modalities, including exposure risk, underlying predisposition, cross-sectional imaging, and direct and/or indirect pancreatic function tests. The first step to diagnose CP is to perform a detailed history to attempt to elucidate underlying risk factors. Key elements that must be investigated are hypertriglyceridemia, autoimmune diseases, diabetes mellitus, and prior AP episodes [68, 69]. The most common clinical manifestations of CP are abdominal pain and steatorrhea depending on the degree of pancreatic dysfunction.

Pain is the dominant symptom of CP. It is usually recurrent and can be either episodic (type A) or persistent (type B). Up to 80–90% of patients complain of pain during the course of the disease. Painless pancreatitis occurs in 10–20% of patients [40, 70–73].

The occurrence, the etiology and the sequalae of prior episodes of AP should be determined. Family history is informative especially in patients with early-onset disease to determine if hereditary or genetic causes are responsible. The use of voluptuous substances such as tobacco and alcohol should be investigated as these are the main driving factors, for example using the AUDIT questionnaire.

Laboratory values should be tested: triglyceride-levels; Ca^{++}-levels for ruling out elevated pHPT; carbohydrate deficient transferrin (CDT)/phosphatidylethanol levels.

The sensitivity of pancreatic function testing to diagnose CP is low. To date, there are no randomized clinical trials, systematic reviews or meta-analysis which specifically address the use of pancreatic function tests to diagnose CP. As such, pancreatic function tests should only be used as ancillary test in making the diagnosis [74–76].

Pancreas has a large reserve and only a significant loss of function (usually >90%) results in the clinically apparent symptoms of vitamin deficiency, steatorrhea and azotorrhea [77]. EPI is the result of the imbalance within nutritional intake, pancreatic digestive enzyme delivery to the small intestine, intestinal adaptation to disease and nutritional needs. CP is an evolving process, and exocrine function is progressively impaired from a reduced functional capacity to exocrine failure in the late phase. To detect mild or moderate exocrine pancreatic impairment, invasive tests employing a hormonal secretagogue (CCK or secretin stimulation tests) maximally stimulating pancreatic secretion can be useful. Such tests are sensitive but poorly specific, they are not diagnostic [78, 79]. Conversely, nonhormonal tests of pancreatic function can detect severe exocrine insufficiency only. Indeed, fecal elastase and fecal chymotrypsin can be used in the follow-up of selected patients for identifying a progressive impairment in pancreatic function by which the chronicity of the inflammatory process can be confirmed [80–82].

It is critical to demonstrate typical morphological changes in the pancreas, as imaging is a surrogate for histology. Diagnosis is established via high quality imaging modalities, which allow identification of the following signs: increased density of the parenchyma, atrophy of the gland, calcification, pseudocysts and irregularities of the main pancreatic duct and its side branches. Diagnosis should be based on imaging performed in symptomatic patients presenting with indicators suggestive of pancreatic disease [29].

MR with MR cholangio-pancreatography and dynamic MRCP following secretin administration and endoscopic ultrasound are the imaging techniques of choice to diagnose early CP and to identify pancreatic malformations in patients with CP. In early CP dynamic MRCP during secretin administration is useful in identifying initial morphological changes of the pancreatic duct system and specifically of the side branches [83].

CT is the technique of choice in diagnosing and localizing pancreatic stones inside the lumen of the main pancreatic duct or side branches, and in patients with CP and flare of the disease [84].

Transabdominal ultrasonography (US) is not able to identify early CP, but can confirm the diagnosis of advanced CP, since it identifies the thinning of the pancreatic parenchyma, the irregularity of the pancreatic margins, dilatation of the main pancreatic duct and of the side branches, and endoductal calcified stones [85].

When the diagnosis cannot be made by radiological or EUS morphologic criteria and clinical and functional evidence of CP is strong, histological examination via EUS-guided fine-needle biopsy is the gold-standard to diagnose CP [36].

Testing for germline mutations is not diagnostic of CP, but it rather identifies a population at risk improving the accuracy of biomarkers and identifies the mechanism underlying the pathogenic process. Therapies can target the mechanism, and knowing the mechanism allow to select the most appropriate drug. Patients should be referred to a genetic counselor for evaluation. At minimum patients with idiopathic CP should be evaluated for PRSS1, SPINK1, CFTR, and CTRC gene mutation analysis.

3.5 Management

3.5.1 Pain

Abdominal pain is the most common complication and prevailing symptom of CP. It can manifest through a spectrum of intensity, form mild and intermittent to severe unrelenting. Pain is experienced by 75% of patients at the time of presentation and up to 97% during the clinical course. The pathophysiology is multifactorial and results from pancreatic and extra-pancreatic causes. Pancreas-related causes include: parenchymal and nerve sheaths inflammatory infiltrates, augmented pressure by obstruction flow of pancreatic juice and increased pancreatic capsule tension due to raised pancreatic parenchymal pressure. Extra-pancreatic causes include gastric or duodenal ulcers and meteorism caused by bacterial overgrowth and maldigestion [47, 86].

The NAPS-2 Study categorized five distinct pain patterns according to severity and pain control (**Table 9**) [87].

The only pain score explicitly validated for assessing pain in patients with CP has been published in 1995 by Bloechle et al. [88]: the visual analogue scale. Pain management should follow the WHO three-step analgesic ladder. However, WHO pain management has not been consistently used in the available literature, thus the question about its effectiveness cannot be answered.

The natural course of pain in CP is characterized by a variable percentage of patients (47–80%) achieving spontaneous pain relief from 10 to 15 years from onset. However, a part of patients will suffer of pain indefinitely. Waiting for a spontaneous pain relief has been defined not reliable by the American Gastroenterological Association (AGA) [36].

Endoscopic treatment (ET) is recommended as a first-choice therapy in patients with an obstructive type of pancreatic pain and in patients with a pancreatic duct dilatation. This could, also, be useful as a bridge to surgery. The aim of ET is decompression of an obstructed main pancreatic duct, it decreases the numbers of hospitalizations for pancreatic pain and reduces analgesics intake. Extracorporeal shock wave lithotripsy (ESWL) therapy in painful CP is indicated if the stone size is >5 mm, the stone is located in the head or pancreatic body, and there are no strictures of the main pancreatic duct. It should be combined with ET in cases of large stones with pancreatic duct stricture [36, 47].

Surgical options for pain are classified into three categories: decompression (focusing on ductal hypertension), resection (focusing on inflammatory masses in the pancreatic head), and mixed techniques. Decompression is recommended in patients with a main pancreatic duct >7–8 mm and no inflammatory mass. Pain relief is achieved in 66–91% of patients, however, the long-term results show up to 50%

Pain pattern	Description
A	I have episodes of mild to moderate pain, usually controlled by medicines
B	I have constant mild to moderate pain, usually controlled by medicines
C	I am usually free of abdominal pain, but I have episodes of severe pain
D	I have constant mild pain that is controlled, plus episodes of severe pain
E	I have constant severe pain that does not change

Table 9.
Description of pain patterns used in the NAPS2 study.

recurrences. Resection in patients with an inflammatory mass or an obstructive CP of the body or tail. Pancreaticoduodenectomy is effective in 75% of patients but with a significant morbidity (20%), as such most authors favor the more conservative mixed techniques. Mixed techniques achieve a short-term pain relief in up to 70–100% of patients and a long-term pain relief in 82–100%. Mixed techniques are based on the resection of the inflammatory mass in the pancreatic head and drainage of the obstructed main pancreatic duct (body and tail). The most widely used techniques are the duodenal preservation (Berger) or the Frey method which consists in a longitudinal pancreaticojejunostomy and in the coring out of the pancreatic head [47, 89].

A pain management strategy must be well structured and conducted with a logical approach to minimize long term complication and sequelae. Is recommended to early involve a pain management specialist during the clinical course, as delays lead to poorer health and pain control [90].

3.5.2 Lifestyle

Complete cessation of alcohol and tobacco use is of utmost importance. Patients must be aware that ongoing use will sustain the cycle of pain and lead to further progression of the disease. Cognitive and mindfulness-based therapies should be offered to all patients, especially for those who need assistance with abuse disorder.

3.5.3 Enzyme replacement

A weight loss of more than 10% of the body weight, steatorrhea with a fecal fat excretion of more than 15 g/die (or a pathological pancreatic function test) in combination with clinical signs of malabsorption (dyspeptic symptoms with severe meteorism or diarrhea) are a clinical indication for pancreatic enzyme replacement therapy. Abdominal complaints (diarrhea/steatorrhea, abdominal distension/meteorism and pain) may be due to intestinal motility disorders caused by maldigestion and malabsorption [91]. Enzyme supplements are administered by gastric-acid-protected encapsulated microsphere and contain pancreatin, with the main components being lipase, amylase, trypsin and chymotrypsin. A successful treatment is measured by improvement of the disease symptoms. Therapy with pancreatin purely as a trial for 4–6 weeks may also be beneficial if symptoms are unclear [91–94].

An untreated severe EPI results in a severe malabsorption syndrome that manifests in the form of steatorrhea, deficiency of fat-soluble vitamins, weight loss and finally cachexia [71, 95, 96]. The success of enzyme replacement therapy should be monitored using clinical parameters (weight gain, long-term normalization of the vitamin status, cessation of abdominal symptoms).

3.6 Surveillance

Incidence of pancreatic cancer is increased in long-lasting CP. Several studies have addressed this topic. The paper by Bansal and Sonnenberg in 1995 found a clear relationship between CP and pancreatic cancer (OR 2.23; 95% CI 1.43–3.49) [97].

Should patients with CP be screened for pancreatic cancer? The United States Preventive Task force has stated that screening the general population for pancreatic cancer by current modalities is not recommended.

4. Surgical treatment of complications

Local complications such as pancreatic and/or peripancreatic fluid collections can occur after an episode of AP or after recrudescence of CP or a blunt, penetrating, iatrogenic pancreatic trauma. Peripancreatic fluid collections, with or without a necrotic component, are early manifestations of the pancreatic inflammatory process.

In asymptomatic patients, clinical observation and periodic imaging follow up represent the most successful management. Prognosis and management are greatly affected by the recognition between sterile and infected pancreatic necrosis. In symptomatic patients, with rapidly enlarging pseudocysts or systemic manifestations of organ failure sustained by an infectious process, an interventional treatment is indicated. In this case endoscopic drainage approach is the first choice, especially when fluid collection is close to gastroduodenal lumen. A combination of techniques is possible in patients with large collections, extended in pelvis and paracolic gutters, or multiple collections [98].

Endoscopic management of pseudocysts and walled-off pancreatic necrosis (WOPN) has been described in a dedicated chapter of this Book.

Endoscopic drainage techniques consist in [99]: *transmural or transpapillary drainage*.

Percutaneous drainage remains an important treatment modality for patients with symptomatic collections. It may be used both as primary therapy and as an adjunct to other techniques. According to the last International [3], American [100] and Japanese [24] guidelines, percutaneous catheter (or endoscopic transmural drainage) should be the first step in the treatment of patients with suspected or confirmed (walled-off) infected necrotizing pancreatitis. This is applied to decompress retroperitoneal fluid collections, to provide a rapid and effective means for source control in patients with infected pancreatic necrosis. The positioning can be performed via the transperitoneal or retroperitoneal approaches. Retroperitoneal route is generally preferred because it avoids peritoneal contamination, enteric fistulas and facilitates a possible step-up approach.

The surgical odyssey in managing necrotizing pancreatitis is a notable example of how evidence-based knowledge leads to improvement in patient care. In the beginning of the 20th century surgeons such as Mayo Robson, Mickulicz, and Moynihan, in the context of the progression of anesthesia, were induced to deploy laparotomy in an effort to treat complications of severe AP [101]. Over the next decades surgical intervention became the therapy of choice despite a mortality rate greater than 50%. Extensive pancreatic resection became the treatment of choice in the 1960s and 1970s. Innovations and increased accuracy in radiological techniques led to new approaches for management. Since 1990s several studies proved that nonoperative management of patients with sterile pancreatic necrosis was superior to surgical intervention, and that delayed intervention provided improved surgical mortality rates. The treatment of infected necrosis shifted to a more conservative approach also thanks to a comprehensive knowledge of the physio-pathological process of the systemic inflammatory response and the adoption of novel antibiotics in curbing systemic toxicity and protecting against organ failure.

According to the last guidelines of the Working Group of the IAP/APA published in 2013 [3] and of the AGA published in 2020 [100], a symptomatic sterile pancreatic necrosis is an indication for intervention (either radiological, endoscopical or surgical). In case of infected pancreatic necrosis invasive procedures (e.g. percutaneous catheter drainage, endoscopic transluminal drainage/necrosectomy, minimally invasive or open necrosectomy) should be delayed, where possible, until at least 4 weeks after initial presentation to permit the collection to become "walled-off".

Percutaneous drainage, alone or in combination with other minimally invasive approaches, can be an effective means for source control in patients with infected pancreatic necrosis. A significant number of patients (23–47%) will resolve their necrosis with percutaneous drainage alone. In those with persistent disease, a step up to operative intervention may be undertaken. The tract of the drain is utilized to access the retroperitoneal space for an intracavitary videoscopic necrosectomy by which drains are left in the cavity for lavage and fistula control [102–104].

Open debridement with external drainage still plays an important, albeit limited, role. After access to retroperitoneum, fluid is evacuated and necrotic dissection and debridement is made. In biliary pancreatitis, cholecystectomy should be practiced but it is associated with increased incidence of postoperative bile leak or biliary injury. Colon resection and colostomy have to be considered if mesocolon is involved in peripancreatic necrosis. A feeding enteral tube and at least two-four drainage tubes should be placed [105].

Each approach has distinct peculiarities with pros and cons that must be weighted in each case planning: pattern of disease, physiology of the patient, expertise of the multidisciplinary team, and the resources of the center [100].

Conflict of interest

The authors declare no conflict of interest.

Author details

Tommaso Stecca*, Cristina Nistri, Bruno Pauletti, Adriana Di Giacomo, Flavio Colaut, Mariangela Ruperto, Ezio Caratozzolo, Luca Bonariol and Marco Massani
Surgery Department, First Surgical Unit, Treviso Regional Hospital, Azienda ULSS2 Marca Trevigiana, Italy

*Address all correspondence to: tommaso.stecca@aulss2.veneto.it

References

[1] Crockett SD, Wani S, Gardner TB, Falck-Ytter Y, Barkun AN. American Gastroenterological Association Institute Guideline on initial management of acute pancreatitis. Gastroenterology. 2018;**154**:1096-1101. DOI: 10.1053/j.gastro.2018.01.032

[2] Leppäniemi A, Tolonen M, Tarasconi A, Segovia-Lohse H, Gamberini E, et al. 2019 WSES guidelines for the management of severe acute pancreatitis. World Journal of Emergency Surgery. 2019;**14**:27. DOI: 10.1186/s13017-019-0247-0

[3] Iap WG, Acute APA, Guidelines P. IAP/APA evidence-based guidelines for the management of acute pancreatitis. Pancreatology. 2013;**13**:1-15. DOI: 10.1016/j.pan.2013.07.063

[4] Ismail OZ, Bhayana V. Lipase or amylase for the diagnosis of acute pancreatitis? Clinical Biochemistry. 2017;**50**:1275-1280. DOI: 10.1016/j.clinbiochem.2017.07.003

[5] Forsmark CE, Vege SS, Wilcox CM. Acute pancreatitis. New England Journal of Medicine. 2016;**375**:1972-1981. DOI: 10.1056/NEJMra1505202

[6] Tenner S, Baillie J, DeWitt J, Vege SS. American College of Gastroenterology guideline: management of acute pancreatitis. American Journal of Gastroenterology. 2013;**108**:1400-1416. DOI: 10.1038/ajg.2013.218

[7] Banks PA, Bollen TL, Dervenis C, Gooszen HG, Johnson CD, et al. Classification of acute pancreatitis - 2012: revision of the Atlanta classification and definitions by international consensus. Gut. 2013;**62**:102-111. DOI: 10.1136/gutjnl-2012-302779

[8] Gress TM, El-Omar E. Revision of the Atlanta classification of acute pancreatitis. Gut. Jan 2013;**62**(1):102-111. DOI: 10.1136/gutjnl-2012-302779. Epub 2012 Oct 25

[9] Marshall JC, Cook DJ, Christou NV, Bernard GR, Sprung CL, et al. Multiple organ dysfunction score: a reliable descriptor of a complex clinical outcome. Critical Care Medicine. 1995;**23**:1638-1652. DOI: 10.1097/00003246-199510000-00007

[10] Mofidi R, Duff MD, Wigmore SJ, Madhavan KK, Garden OJ, et al. Association between early systemic inflammatory response, severity of multiorgan dysfunction and death in acute pancreatitis. The British Journal of Surgery. 2006;**93**:738-744. DOI: 10.1002/bjs.5290

[11] Singh VK, Wu BU, Bollen TL, Repas K, Maurer R, et al. Early systemic inflammatory response syndrome is associated with severe acute pancreatitis. Clinical Gastroenterology and Hepatology. 2009;**7**:1247-1251. DOI: 10.1016/j.cgh.2009.08.012

[12] Khanna AK, Meher S, Prakash S, Tiwary SK, Singh U, et al. Comparison of Ranson, Glasgow, MOSS, SIRS, BISAP, APACHE-II, CTSI scores, IL-6, CRP, and procalcitonin in predicting severity, organ failure, pancreatic necrosis, and mortality in acute pancreatitis. HPB Surgery: A World Journal of Hepatic, Pancreatic and Biliary Surgery. 2013;**2013**:367581. DOI: 10.1155/2013/367581

[13] Gurda-Duda A, Kuśnierz-Cabala B, Nowak W, Naskalski JW, Kulig J. Assessment of the prognostic value of certain acute-phase proteins and procalcitonin in the prognosis of acute

pancreatitis. Pancreas. 2008;**37**:449-453. DOI: 10.1097/MPA.0b013e3181706d67

[14] Staubli SM, Oertli D, Nebiker CA. Laboratory markers predicting severity of acute pancreatitis. Critical Reviews in Clinical Laboratory Sciences. 2015;**52**: 273-283. DOI: 10.3109/10408363. 2015.1051659

[15] Ranson JH, Rifkind KM, Roses DF, Fink SD, Eng K, et al. Prognostic signs and the role of operative management in acute pancreatitis. Surgery, Gynecology & Obstetrics. 1974;**139**:69-81

[16] Blamey SL, Imrie CW, O'Neill J, Gilmour WH, Carter DC. Prognostic factors in acute pancreatitis. Gut. 1984; **25**:1340-1346. DOI: 10.1136/ gut.25.12.1340

[17] Knaus WA, Draper EA, Wagner DP, Zimmerman JE. APACHE II: a severity of disease classification system. Critical Care Medicine. 1985;**13**:818-829

[18] Le Gall JR, Loirat P, Alperovitch A, Glaser P, Granthil C, et al. A simplified acute physiology score for ICU patients. Critical Care Medicine. 1984;**12**:975-977. DOI: 10.1097/00003246-198411000-00012

[19] Balthazar EJ, Robinson DL, Megibow AJ, Ranson JH. Acute pancreatitis: value of CT in establishing prognosis. Radiology. 1990;**174**:331-336. DOI: 10.1148/radiology.174.2.2296641

[20] Balthazar EJ. Acute pancreatitis: assessment of severity with clinical and CT evaluation. Radiology. 2002;**223**: 603-613. DOI: 10.1148/radiol.2233 010680

[21] Wu BU, Johannes RS, Sun X, Tabak Y, Conwell DL, et al. The early prediction of mortality in acute pancreatitis: a large population-based study. Gut. 2008;**57**:1698-1703. DOI: 10.1136/gut.2008.152702

[22] Lankisch PG, Weber-Dany B, Hebel K, Maisonneuve P, Lowenfels AB. The harmless acute pancreatitis score: a clinical algorithm for rapid initial stratification of nonsevere disease. Clinical Gastroenterology and Hepatology. 2009;**7**:702-705; quiz 607. DOI: 10.1016/j.cgh.2009.02.020

[23] Adam F, Bor C, Uyar M, Demırağ K, Çankayalı İ. Severe acute pancreatitis admitted to intensive care unit: SOFA is superior to Ranson's criteria and APACHE II in determining prognosis. The Turkish Journal of Gastroenterology. 2013;**24**:430-435. DOI: 10.4318/tjg.2013.0761

[24] Isaji S, Takada T, Kawarada Y, Hirata K, Mayumi T, et al. JPN guidelines for the management of acute pancreatitis: surgical management. Journal of Hepato-Biliary-Pancreatic Surgery. 2006;**13**:48-55. DOI: 10.1007/ s00534-005-1051-7

[25] Papachristou GI, Muddana V, Yadav D, O'Connell M, Sanders MK, et al. Comparison of BISAP, Ranson's, APACHE-II, and CTSI scores in predicting organ failure, complications, and mortality in acute pancreatitis. American Journal of Gastroenterology. 2010;**105**:435-441; quiz 442. DOI: 10.1038/ajg.2009.622

[26] Mourad MM, Evans R, Kalidindi V, Navaratnam R, Dvorkin L, et al. Prophylactic antibiotics in acute pancreatitis: endless debate. Annals of the Royal College of Surgeons of England. 2017;**99**:107-112. DOI: 10.1308/ rcsann.2016.0355

[27] Kambhampati S, Park W, Habtezion A. Pharmacologic therapy for acute pancreatitis. World Journal of

Gastroenterology. 2014;**20**:16868-16880. DOI: 10.3748/wjg.v20.i45.16868

[28] Moggia E, Koti R, Belgaumkar AP, Fazio F, Pereira SP, et al. Pharmacological interventions for acute pancreatitis. The Cochrane Database of Systematic Reviews. 2017;**4**:CD011384. DOI: 10.1002/14651858.CD011384.pub2

[29] Petrov MS, Yadav D. Global epidemiology and holistic prevention of pancreatitis. Nature Reviews Gastroenterology & Hepatology. 2019; **16**:175-184. DOI: 10.1038/s41575-018-0087-5

[30] Whitcomb DC, Frulloni L, Garg P, Greer JB, Schneider A, et al. Chronic pancreatitis: an international draft consensus proposal for a new mechanistic definition. Pancreatology. 2016;**16**:218-224. DOI: 10.1016/j.pan.2016.02.001

[31] Whitcomb DC. Peering into the 'Black Box' of the complex chronic pancreatitis syndrome. Pancreas. 2016; **45**:1361-1364. DOI: 10.1097/MPA.0000000000000715

[32] Yadav D, Muddana V, O'Connell M. Hospitalizations for chronic pancreatitis in Allegheny County, Pennsylvania, USA. Pancreatology. 2011;**11**:546–552. DOI: 10.1159/000331498

[33] Lévy P, Domínguez-Muñoz E, Imrie C, Löhr M, Maisonneuve P. Epidemiology of chronic pancreatitis: burden of the disease and consequences. United European Gastroenterology Journal. 2014;**2**:345-354. DOI: 10.1177/2050640614548208

[34] Xiao AY, Tan MLY, Wu LM, Asrani VM, Windsor JA, et al. Global incidence and mortality of pancreatic diseases: a systematic review, meta-analysis, and meta-regression of population-based cohort studies. Lancet Gastroenterology & Hepatology. 2016;**1**: 45-55. DOI: 10.1016/S2468-1253(16)30004-8

[35] Olesen SS, Mortensen LH, Zinck E, Becker U, Drewes AM, et al. Time trends in incidence and prevalence of chronic pancreatitis: a 25-year population-based nationwide study. United European Gastroenterology Journal. 2021;**9**:82-90. DOI: 10.1177/2050640620966513

[36] Gardner TB, Adler DG, Forsmark CE, Sauer BG, Taylor JR, et al. ACG clinical guideline: chronic pancreatitis. American Journal of Gastroenterology. 2020;**115**:322-339. DOI: 10.14309/ajg.0000000000000535

[37] Löhr JM, Dominguez-Munoz E, Rosendahl J, Besselink M, Mayerle J, et al. United European Gastroenterology evidence-based guidelines for the diagnosis and therapy of chronic pancreatitis (HaPanEU). United European Gastroenterol J. 2017;**5**: 153-199. DOI: 10.1177/2050640616684695

[38] Lévy P, Mathurin P, Roqueplo A, Rueff B, Bernades P. A multidimensional case-control study of dietary, alcohol, and tobacco habits in alcoholic men with chronic pancreatitis. Pancreas. 1995;**10**: 231-238. DOI: 10.1097/00006676-199504000-00003

[39] Guyatt GH, Oxman AD, Vist GE, Kunz R, Falck-Ytter Y, et al. GRADE: an emerging consensus on rating quality of evidence and strength of recommendations. BMJ. 2008;**336**: 924-926. DOI: 10.1136/bmj.39489.470347.AD

[40] Witt H, Apte MV, Keim V, Wilson JS. Chronic pancreatitis: challenges and advances in pathogenesis, genetics, diagnosis, and therapy.

Gastroenterology. 2007;**132**:1557-1573. DOI: 10.1053/j.gastro.2007.03.001

[41] Maisonneuve P, Lowenfels AB, Müllhaupt B, Cavallini G, Lankisch PG, et al. Cigarette smoking accelerates progression of alcoholic chronic pancreatitis. Gut. 2005;**54**:510-514. DOI: 10.1136/gut.2004.039263

[42] Ammann RW, Knoblauch M, Möhr P, Deyhle P, Largiadèr F, et al. High incidence of extrapancreatic carcinoma in chronic pancreatitis. Scandinavian Journal of Gastroenterology. 1980;**15**:395-399. DOI: 10.3109/00365528009181490

[43] Ammann RW, Muellhaupt B. The natural history of pain in alcoholic chronic pancreatitis. Gastroenterology. 1999;**116**:1132-1140. DOI: 10.1016/s0016-5085(99)70016-8

[44] Yadav D, Hawes RH, Brand RE, Anderson MA, Money ME, et al. Alcohol consumption, cigarette smoking, and the risk of recurrent acute and chronic pancreatitis. Archives of Internal Medicine. 2009;**169**:1035-1045. DOI: 10.1001/archinternmed.2009.125

[45] Jacob JJ, John M, Thomas N, Chacko A, Cherian R, et al. Does hyperparathyroidism cause pancreatitis? A South Indian experience and a review of published work. ANZ Journal of Surgery. 2006;**76**:740-744. DOI: 10.1111/j.1445-2197.2006.03845.x

[46] Carnaille B, Oudar C, Pattou F, Combemale F, Rocha J, et al. Pancreatitis and primary hyperparathyroidism: forty cases. The Australian and New Zealand Journal of Surgery. 1998;**68**:117-119. DOI: 10.1111/j.1445-2197.1998.tb04719.x

[47] Hoffmeister A, Mayerle J, Beglinger C, Büchler MW, Bufler P, et al. English language version of the S3-consensus guidelines on chronic pancreatitis: definition, aetiology, diagnostic examinations, medical, endoscopic and surgical management of chronic pancreatitis. Zeitschrift Fur Gastroenterologie. 2015;**53**:1447-1495. DOI: 10.1055/s-0041-107379

[48] Whitcomb DC. Primer on precision medicine for complex chronic disorders. Clinical and Translational Gastroenterology. 2019;**10**:e00067. DOI: 10.14309/ctg.0000000000000067

[49] Whitcomb DC, Gorry MC, Preston RA, Furey W, Sossenheimer MJ, et al. Hereditary pancreatitis is caused by a mutation in the cationic trypsinogen gene. Nature Genetics. 1996;**14**:141-145. DOI: 10.1038/ng1096-141

[50] Witt H, Luck W, Hennies HC, Classen M, Kage A, et al. Mutations in the gene encoding the serine protease inhibitor, Kazal type 1 are associated with chronic pancreatitis. Nature Genetics. 2000;**25**:213-216. DOI: 10.1038/76088

[51] Sharer N, Schwarz M, Malone G, Howarth A, Painter J, et al. Mutations of the cystic fibrosis gene in patients with chronic pancreatitis. The New England Journal of Medicine. 1998;**339**:645-652. DOI: 10.1056/NEJM199809033391001

[52] Rosendahl J, Witt H, Szmola R, Bhatia E, Ozsvári B, et al. Chymotrypsin C (CTRC) variants that diminish activity or secretion are associated with chronic pancreatitis. Nature Genetics. 2008;**40**:78-82. DOI: 10.1038/ng.2007.44

[53] Witt H, Beer S, Rosendahl J, Chen J-M, Chandak GR, et al. Variants in CPA1 are strongly associated with early onset chronic pancreatitis. Nature Genetics. 2013;**45**:1216-1220. DOI: 10.1038/ng.2730

[54] Fjeld K, Weiss FU, Lasher D, Rosendahl J, Chen J-M, et al. A recombined allele of the lipase gene CEL and its pseudogene CELP confers susceptibility to chronic pancreatitis. Nature Genetics. 2015;**47**:518-522. DOI: 10.1038/ng.3249

[55] Howes N, Lerch MM, Greenhalf W, Stocken DD, Ellis I, et al. Clinical and genetic characteristics of hereditary pancreatitis in Europe. Clinical Gastroenterology and Hepatology. 2004; **2**:252-261. DOI: 10.1016/s1542-3565(04) 00013-8

[56] Applebaum-Shapiro SE, Finch R, Pfützer RH, Hepp LA, Gates L, et al. Hereditary pancreatitis in North America: the Pittsburgh-Midwest Multi-Center Pancreatic Study Group Study. Pancreatology. 2001;**1**:439-443. DOI: 10.1159/000055844

[57] Rebours V, Boutron-Ruault M-C, Jooste V, Bouvier A-M, Hammel P, et al. Mortality rate and risk factors in patients with hereditary pancreatitis: uni- and multidimensional analyses. American Journal of Gastroenterology. 2009;**104**: 2312-2317. DOI: 10.1038/ajg.2009.363

[58] Le Bodic L, Schnee M, Georgelin T, Soulard F, Ferec C, et al. An exceptional genealogy for hereditary chronic pancreatitis. Digestive Diseases and Sciences. 1996;**41**:1504-1510. DOI: 10.1007/BF02088580

[59] Yatto RP, Siegel JH. The role of pancreatobiliary duct anatomy in the etiology of alcoholic pancreatitis. Journal of Clinical Gastroenterology. 1984;**6**: 419-423. DOI: 10.1097/ 00004836-198410000-00005

[60] Whitcomb DC, Preston RA, Aston CE, Sossenheimer MJ, Barua PS, et al. A gene for hereditary pancreatitis maps to chromosome 7q35. Gastroenterology. 1996;**110**:1975-1980. DOI: 10.1053/gast.1996.v110.pm896 4426

[61] Sarles H, Sarles JC, Muratore R, Guien C. Chronic inflammatory sclerosis of the pancreas - an autonomous pancreatic disease? The American Journal of Digestive Diseases. 1961;**6**: 688-698. DOI: 10.1007/BF02232341

[62] Yoshida K, Toki F, Takeuchi T, Watanabe S, Shiratori K, et al. Chronic pancreatitis caused by an autoimmune abnormality. Proposal of the concept of autoimmune pancreatitis. Digestive Diseases and Sciences. 1995;**40**: 1561-1568. DOI: 10.1007/BF02285209

[63] Chari ST. Diagnosis of autoimmune pancreatitis using its five cardinal features: introducing the Mayo Clinic's HISORt criteria. Journal of Gastroenterology. 2007;**42**:39-41. DOI: 10.1007/s00535-007-2046-8

[64] Chari ST, Smyrk TC, Levy MJ, Topazian MD, Takahashi N, et al. Diagnosis of autoimmune pancreatitis: the Mayo Clinic experience. Clinical Gastroenterology and Hepatology. 2006; **4**:1010-1016; quiz 934. DOI: 10.1016/ j.cgh.2006.05.017

[65] Kamisawa T, Egawa N, Nakajima H, Tsuruta K, Okamoto A, et al. Clinical difficulties in the differentiation of autoimmune pancreatitis and pancreatic carcinoma. American Journal of Gastroenterology. 2003;**98**:2694-2699. DOI: 10.1111/j.1572-0241.2003.08775.x

[66] Chari ST, Kloeppel G, Zhang L, Notohara K, Lerch MM, et al. Histopathologic and clinical subtypes of autoimmune pancreatitis: the Honolulu consensus document. Pancreas. 2010;**39**: 549-554. DOI: 10.1097/MPA.0b013e3181 e4d9e5

[67] Schneider A, Löhr JM, Mv S. The M-ANNHEIM classification of chronic pancreatitis: Introduction of a unifying classification system based on a review of previous classifications of the disease. Journal of Gastroenterology. 2007;**42**: 101-119. DOI: 10.1007/s00535-006-1945-4

[68] Whitcomb DC. Pancreatitis: TIGAR-O version 2 risk/etiology checklist with topic reviews, updates, and use primers. Clinical and Translational Gastroenterology. 2019;**10**: e1-e14. DOI: 10.14309/ctg.00000 00000000027

[69] Singh VK, Yadav D, Garg PK. Diagnosis and management of chronic pancreatitis: a review. JAMA - Journal of the American Medical Association. 2019; **322**:2422-2434. DOI: 10.1001/ jama.2019.19411

[70] Warshaw AL, Banks PA, Fernández-Del CC. AGA technical review: treatment of pain in chronic pancreatitis. Gastroenterology. 1998;**115**:765-776. DOI: 10.1016/s0016-5085(98)70157-x

[71] Layer P, Yamamoto H, Kalthoff L, Clain JE, Bakken LJ, et al. The different courses of early- and late-onset idiopathic and alcoholic chronic pancreatitis. Gastroenterology. 1994;**107**: 1481-1487. DOI: 10.1016/0016-5085(94) 90553-3

[72] Vege SS, Chari ST. Chronic pancreatitis. The New England Journal of Medicine. 2022;**386**:869-878. DOI: 10.1056/NEJMcp1809396

[73] Wang LW, Li ZS, Li S De, Jin ZD, Zou DW, et al. Prevalence and clinical features of chronic pancreatitis in China: a retrospective multicenter analysis over 10 years. Pancreas. 2009;**38**:248–254. DOI:10.1097/MPA.0b013e31818f6ac1

[74] Conwell DL, Lee LS, Yadav D, Longnecker DS, Miller FH, et al. American Pancreatic Association practice guidelines in chronic pancreatitis evidence-based report on diagnostic guidelines. Pancreas. 2014;**43**: 1143-1162. DOI: 10.1097/MPA.0000 000000000237

[75] Ramesh H. Proposal for a new grading system for chronic pancreatitis: the ABC system. Journal of Clinical Gastroenterology. 2002;**35**:67-70. DOI: 10.1097/00004836-200207000-00014

[76] Bagul A, Siriwardena AK. Evaluation of the Manchester classification system for chronic pancreatitis. JOP: Journal of the Pancreas. 2006;**7**:390-396

[77] DiMagno EP, Go VL. Exocrine pancreatic insufficiency. Current concepts of pathophysiology. Postgraduate Medicine. 1972;**52**:135-140. DOI: 10.1080/00325481.1972.11713185

[78] Chowdhury RS, Forsmark CE. Review article: pancreatic function testing. Alimentary Pharmacology & Therapeutics. 2003;**17**:733-750. DOI: 10.1046/j.1365-2036.2003.01495.x

[79] Niederau C, Grendell JH. Diagnosis of chronic pancreatitis. Gastroenterology. 1985;**88**:1973-1995. DOI: 10.1016/ 0016-5085(85)90029-0

[80] Lankisch PG, Schmidt I, König H, Lehnick D, Knollmann R, et al. Faecal elastase 1: not helpful in diagnosing chronic pancreatitis associated with mild to moderate exocrine pancreatic insufficiency. Gut. 1998;**42**:551-554. DOI: 10.1136/gut.42.4.551

[81] Naruse S, Ishiguro H, Ko SBH, Yoshikawa T, Yamamoto T, et al. Fecal pancreatic elastase: a reproducible marker for severe exocrine pancreatic

insufficiency. Journal of Gastroenterology. 2006;**41**:901-908. DOI: 10.1007/s00535-006-1884-0

[82] Symersky T, van der Zon A, Biemond I, Masclee AA. Faecal elastase-I: helpful in analysing steatorrhoea? The Netherlands Journal of Medicine. 2004; **62**:286-289

[83] Manfredi R, Costamagna G, Vecchioli A, Colagrande C, Spina S, et al. Dynamic pancreatography with magnetic resonance after functional stimulus with secretin in chronic pancreatitis. La Radiologia medica. 1998; **96**:226-231

[84] Kamat R, Gupta P, Rana S. Imaging in chronic pancreatitis: state of the art review. The Indian Journal of Radiology & Imaging. 2019;**29**:201-210. DOI: 10.4103/ijri.IJRI_484_18

[85] Etemad B, Whitcomb DC. Chronic pancreatitis: diagnosis, classification, and new genetic developments. Gastroenterology. 2001;**120**:682-707. DOI: 10.1053/gast.2001.22586

[86] Kichler A, Jang S. Chronic pancreatitis: epidemiology, diagnosis, and management updates. Drugs. 2020; **80**:1155-1168. DOI: 10.1007/s40265-020-01360-6

[87] Whitcomb DC, Yadav D, Adam S, Hawes RH, Brand RE, et al. Multicenter approach to recurrent acute and chronic pancreatitis in the United States: the North American Pancreatitis Study 2 (NAPS2). Pancreatology. 2008;**8**: 520-531. DOI: 10.1159/000152001

[88] Bloechle C, Izbicki JR, Knoefel WT, Kuechler T, Broelsch CE. Quality of life in chronic pancreatitis - results after duodenum-preserving resection of the head of the pancreas. Pancreas. 1995;**11**: 77-85. DOI: 10.1097/00006676-199507000-00008

[89] Frulloni L, Falconi M, Gabbrielli A, Gaia E, Graziani R, et al. Italian consensus guidelines for chronic pancreatitis. Digestive and Liver Disease. 2010;**42**:S381-S406. DOI: 10.1016/S1590-8658(10)60682-2

[90] Drewes AM, Bouwense SAW, Campbell CM, Ceyhan GO, Delhaye M, et al. Guidelines for the understanding and management of pain in chronic pancreatitis. Pancreatology. 2017;**17**: 720-731. DOI: 10.1016/j.pan.2017.07.006

[91] Layer P, von der Ohe MR, Holst JJ, Jansen JB, Grandt D, et al. Altered postprandial motility in chronic pancreatitis: role of malabsorption. Gastroenterology. 1997;**112**:1624-1634. DOI: 10.1016/s0016-5085(97)70045-3

[92] Regan PT, Malagelada JR, DiMagno EP, Glanzman SL, Go VL. Comparative effects of antacids, cimetidine and enteric coating on the therapeutic response to oral enzymes in severe pancreatic insufficiency. The New England Journal of Medicine. 1977;**297**: 854-858. DOI: 10.1056/NEJM197710202971603

[93] Wooldridge JL, Heubi JE, Amaro-Galvez R, Boas SR, Blake KV, et al. EUR-1008 pancreatic enzyme replacement is safe and effective in patients with cystic fibrosis and pancreatic insufficiency. Journal of Cystic Fibrosis: Official Journal of the European Cystic Fibrosis Society. 2009;**8**:405-417. DOI: 10.1016/j.jcf.2009.07.006

[94] Meier R, Ockenga J, Pertkiewicz M, Pap A, Milinic N, et al. ESPEN guidelines on enteral nutrition: pancreas. Clinical Nutrition (Edinburgh, Scotland). 2006; **25**:275-284. DOI: 10.1016/j.clnu.2006.01.019

[95] DiMagno EP, Malagelada JR, Go VL, Moertel CG. Fate of orally ingested enzymes in pancreatic insufficiency. Comparison of two dosage schedules. The New England Journal of Medicine. 1977;**296**:1318-1322. DOI: 10.1056/NEJM197706092962304

[96] DiMagno EP, Go VL, Summerskill WH. Relations between pancreatic enzyme outputs and malabsorption in severe pancreatic insufficiency. The New England Journal of Medicine. 1973;**288**:813-815. DOI: 10.1056/NEJM197304192881603

[97] Bansal P, Sonnenberg A. Pancreatitis is a risk factor for pancreatic cancer. Gastroenterology. 1995;**109**: 247-251. DOI: 10.1016/0016-5085(95)90291-0

[98] Werner J, Feuerbach S, Uhl W, Büchler MW. Management of acute pancreatitis: From surgery to interventional intensive care. Gut. Mar 2005;**54**(3):426-436. DOI: 10.1136/gut.2003.035907

[99] Binmoeller KF, Seifert H, Walter A, Soehendra N. Transpapillary and transmural drainage of pancreatic pseudocysts. Gastrointestinal Endoscopy. Sep 1995;**42**(3): 219-224. DOI: 10.1016/S0016-5107(95)70095-1

[100] Baron TH, DiMaio CJ, Wang AY, Morgan KA. American gastroenterological association clinical practice update: Management of pancreatic necrosis. Gastroenterology. Jan 2020;**158**(1):67-75.e1. DOI: 10.1053/j.gastro.2019.07.064

[101] Bradley EL, Dexter ND. Management of severe acute pancreatitis: A surgical odyssey. Annals of Surgery. Jan 2010;**251**(1):6-17. DOI: 10.1097/SLA.0b013e3181c72b79

[102] van Santvoort HC, Besselink MG, Bakker OJ, Hofker HS, Boermeester MA, et al. A step-up approach or open necrosectomy for necrotizing pancreatitis. New England Journal of Medicine. 22 Apr 2010;**362**(16): 1491-1502. DOI: 10.1056/NEJMoa0908821

[103] Horvath K, Freeny P, Escallon J, Heagerty P, Comstock B, et al. Safety and efficacy of video-assisted retroperitoneal debridement for infected pancreatic collections: A multicenter, prospective, single-arm phase 2 study. Archives of Surgery. Sep 2010;**145**(9):817-825. DOI: 10.1001/archsurg.2010.178

[104] Freeny PC, Hauptmann E, Althaus SJ, Traverso LW, Sinanan M. Percutaneous CT-guided catheter drainage of infected acute necrotizing pancreatitis: Techniques and results. American Journal of Roentgenology. Apr 1998;**170**(4):969-975. DOI: 10.2214/ajr.170.4.9530046

[105] Uhl W, Warshaw A, Imrie C, Bassi C, McKay CJ, et al. IAP guidelines for the surgical management of acute pancreatitis. Pancreatology. 2002;**2**(6): 565-573. DOI: 10.1159/000071269

Section 2

Radiologic Features

Chapter 2

Imaging of Pancreatitis

Giovanni Morana, Alessandro Beleù, Francesca Nistri and Silvia Venturini

Abstract

Imaging of pancreatitis is very complicated. Correct detection of the various forms of pancreatitis is essential for adequate early therapy. In acute pancreatitis, imaging is useful for diagnosis, but above all for the research of causes and any complications. In autoimmune forms, imaging raises clinical suspicion and guides the response to therapy and the search for associated pathologies. In chronic pancreatitis, imaging is essential for grading, differential diagnosis with neoplastic diseases and follow-up. The classical CT and MRI methods play a fundamental role in this sense, being increasingly supported by modern special techniques such as S-MRCP and T1-mapping. Finally, interventional radiology today represents one of the main minimally invasive methods for the diagnosis and treatment of complications.

Keywords: pancreatitis, CT, MRI, radiology, MRCP

1. Introduction

Imaging of pancreatitis is complex and requires in-depth knowledge of both radiological techniques and pathophysiology, pathology and clinical manifestation of these diseases. In fact, pancreatitis has very different forms and manifestations, which require completely different treatments, therefore imaging, especially CT and MRI, are fundamental for the early classification and the consequent therapy. Furthermore, many forms of pancreatitis enter into differential diagnoses with other non-inflammatory conditions of the pancreas, for which a correct diagnosis as early as possible is essential. In this chapter, we will analyze the imaging aspects of acute pancreatitis, chronic pancreatitis and rarer forms such as autoimmune and paraduodenal.

2. Acute pancreatitis

Acute pancreatitis (AP) is an acute inflammatory condition with a range of severity and various local and systemic complications. The main etiologies are the presence of gallstones or alcohol abuse (75–80%); other causes are pancreatic tumors, traumatic or iatrogenic damage and drugs (thiazide diuretics, steroids, azathioprine). In 10–15% of patients, the cause is not identified [1].

The 2012 Revised Atlanta Criteria is an update of the 1992 original classification of AP and is aimed to clarify and improve the terminology of severity grading and local complications. AP is now divided into two distinct subtypes based on the presence or the absence of parenchymal necrosis: necrotizing pancreatitis (NP) and interstitial edematous pancreatitis (IEP). Patients can develop four distinct collection subtypes that are identified based on the presence of pancreatic necrosis and the time elapsed since the pancreatitis onset (with 4 weeks as a threshold). Acute peripancreatic fluid collections (APFCs; <4 weeks) and pseudocysts (PSCs: >4 weeks) occur in IEP and contain fluid only. Acute necrotic collections (ANCs; <4 weeks) and walled-off necrosis (WONs: >4 weeks) occur only in NP and contain fluid with necrotic debris. APFCs and ANCs are acute complications and they may either resolve or persist, developing a mature wall to become delayed complications such as PSCs or WONs, respectively. In addition, any collection subtypes may become infected and may lead to other local or systemic complications [2, 3].

The pancreatitis severity scale has also been updated to improve the stratification and the management of patients; to the original categories of mild and severe AP, based on the presence of organ failure, a third moderately severe AP category has been added for patients with local complications, substantial morbidity and low mortality. A variety of imaging-based scoring systems can be applied to predict severity although they do not account for risk factors like obesity. The computed tomography severity index (CTSI) is the most commonly used and recommended scoring system, it combines the Balthazar grade with the extent of the pancreatic necrosis on a 10-point severity scale as shown in **Table 1**.

Radiological examinations offer various imaging modalities which play specific roles in the different phases of acute pancreatitis. In the early phase, during the first week after onset, imaging aims to establish the diagnosis, determine the etiology and stage the severity; in the late phase, imaging is needed to establish and monitor complications and to guide interventional procedures.

2.1 Imaging in the early phase

The onset of pancreatitis is considered to coincide with the first day of pain; in the first week after onset, the imaging findings correlate poorly with the clinical severity, but they may be useful in assessing the cause of acute pancreatitis [1].

The 2012 Revised Atlanta Classification requires two or more of the following criteria to make a diagnosis of AP: a) abdominal pain suggestive of pancreatitis, b)

Pancreatic features	Balthazar grade	CTSI 0–3 = mild 4–6 = moderate 7–10 = severe
Normal gland	A	0
Local or diffuse swelling	B	1
Peripancreatic fat stranding	C	2
Single acute fluid collection	D	3
≥ 2 acute fluid collections	E	4
No necrosis		0
<30% of necrosis		2
30–50% of necrosis		4
>50% of necrosis		6

Table 1.
Imaging-based scoring systems.

serum amylase or lipase level greater than three times the upper normal value, c) characteristic imaging findings.

Thus, imaging in the initial diagnosis of AP is requested only if the other criteria are not conclusive for the diagnosis but is still necessary in the assessment of the cause of AP.

Ultrasound (US) is the primary imaging technique for the assessment of the biliary tract and should be performed in every patient to rule out gallstones; the examination can also show pancreatic swelling, dilatation of the pancreatic duct or secondary findings like gallbladder or choledochal wall thickening, pericholecystic fluid or fat stranding. The major disadvantage of US is the limited visibility of the pancreatic region because of the presence of overlying bowel gas; moreover, US is poorly accurate in delineating extra pancreatic inflammatory spread and in detecting intrapancreatic necrosis [4, 5].

The American College of Gastroenterology and the American College of Radiology appropriateness criteria recommend performing contrast-enhanced computed tomography or magnetic resonance imaging only in patients with an unclear diagnosis or who do not improve within 48–72 hours of admission [1]. In fact, early CT is indicated if a complication is suspected, even if parenchymal necrosis may be misdiagnosed due to edema and vasoconstriction. The use of a contrast medium is essential for detecting parenchymal necrosis and vascular complications; the standard examination includes an unenhanced phase, a pancreatic phase (delay of 40–50 s) and a portal venous phase (delay of 60–70 s). A monophasic CT protocol is usually sufficient for the diagnosis and the progression assessment, while dual-phase studies (arterial and portal venous) are recommended in case of suspicion of hemorrhage, mesenteric ischemia or arterial pseudoaneurysm or pancreatic mass [3, 5, 6]. In IEP imaging shows a focal or diffuse pancreatic enlargement and an entire parenchymal enhancement with no unenhanced areas (**Figure 1**), although enhancement may be less avid than that of the normal pancreas due to the interstitial edema.

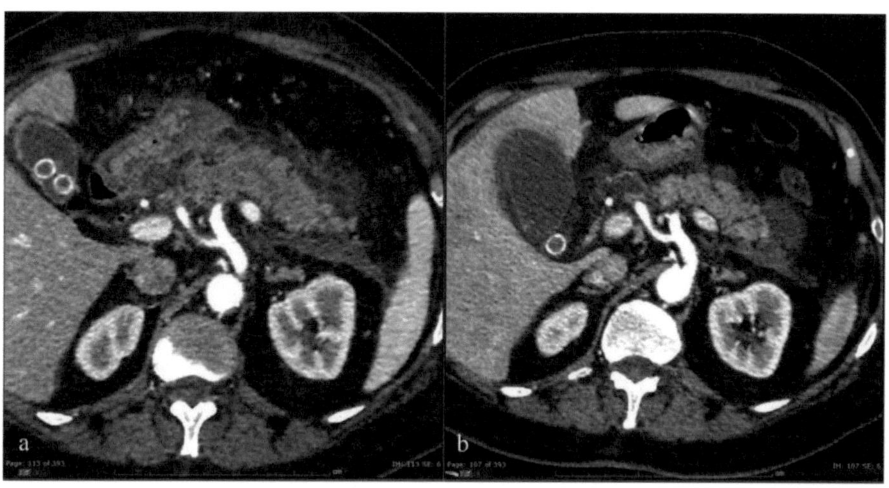

Figure 1.
F, 64 yo, affected by an acute interstitial edematous pancreatitis; At CT a homogeneous decreased enhancement of the entire pancreas is appreciable with no evidence of non-enhancing areas (a); at the level of the tail, a peripancreatic collection is noticeable (b).

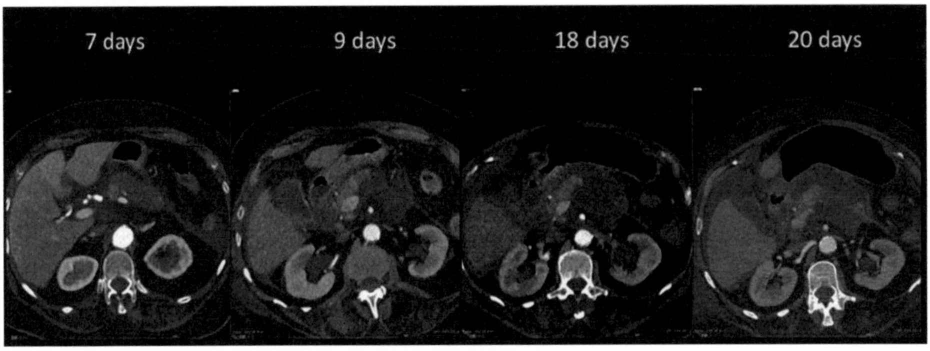

Figure 2.
F, 78 yo, affected by a biliary NP. The patient underwent a CT follow-up that showed a progressive lack of enhancement in the body-tail of the pancreas with large necrotic collections.

Necrotizing pancreatitis (NP) account for 5–10% of all AP and in the early phase, pancreas can appear edematous and hypoenhancing like in IEP, then non-enhancing areas appear as a sign of pancreatic necrosis, which evolves over time (**Figure 2**). There are three subtypes of NP based on the distribution of the necrotic areas: pancreatic NP (5%) without peripancreatic collections, peripancreatic NP (20%) showing peripancreatic necrosis with collections of fluid and components, combined NP (75%) characterized by non-enhancing pancreatic areas and heterogeneous peripancreatic collections [1]. The different subtypes of NP can be observed in the same patient at different times (**Figure 2**).

CT shows the extension of the inflammatory process, but it has a limited capability of differentiating homogeneous fluid collection from debris within collections; moreover, CT has a limited capability of differentiating small necrotic areas from local effusions or focal adipose depositions in elderly people [7].

MRI is an alternative imaging technique especially indicated in case of renal failure, young patients and pregnant women; it is superior to CT in the characterization of pancreatic collections identifying the presence of debris or necrotic material, although its longer scanning time makes its use difficult in uncooperative patients. Moreover, it is useful in the diagnosis of AP when other criteria are inconclusive and US is still uncertain, thanks to its superior sensitivity to pancreatic edema (**Figure 3**). MRI, especially with cholangiopancreatography (MRCP) shows high sensitivity and specificity for choledocholithiasis or congenital anomalies which can explain the AP.

MRI features of IEP include a slight parenchymal hypointensity on T1WI and hyperintensity on T2WI. There may be acute peripancreatic fluid collections showing patchy-like hyperintensity on T2WI in the peripancreatic region, pararenal spaces and lesser omental bursa. Diffusion-weighted imaging (DWI) technique allows a better appreciation of slight pancreatic edema (**Figure 3**).

After contrast agent administration, the pancreas shows homogeneous enhancement. In NP the necrotic areas are hypointense on T1WI, hyperintense on T2WI and have no enhancement after contrast medium. Collections around the pancreas show mixed intensity on T1WI and T2WI, but no enhancement [3, 8].

2.2 Imaging in the late phase: follow up and complications

Imaging is most useful if performed 5–7 days after the onset of AP, when pancreatic necrosis, collections and local complications are distinguishable. The Revised Atlanta

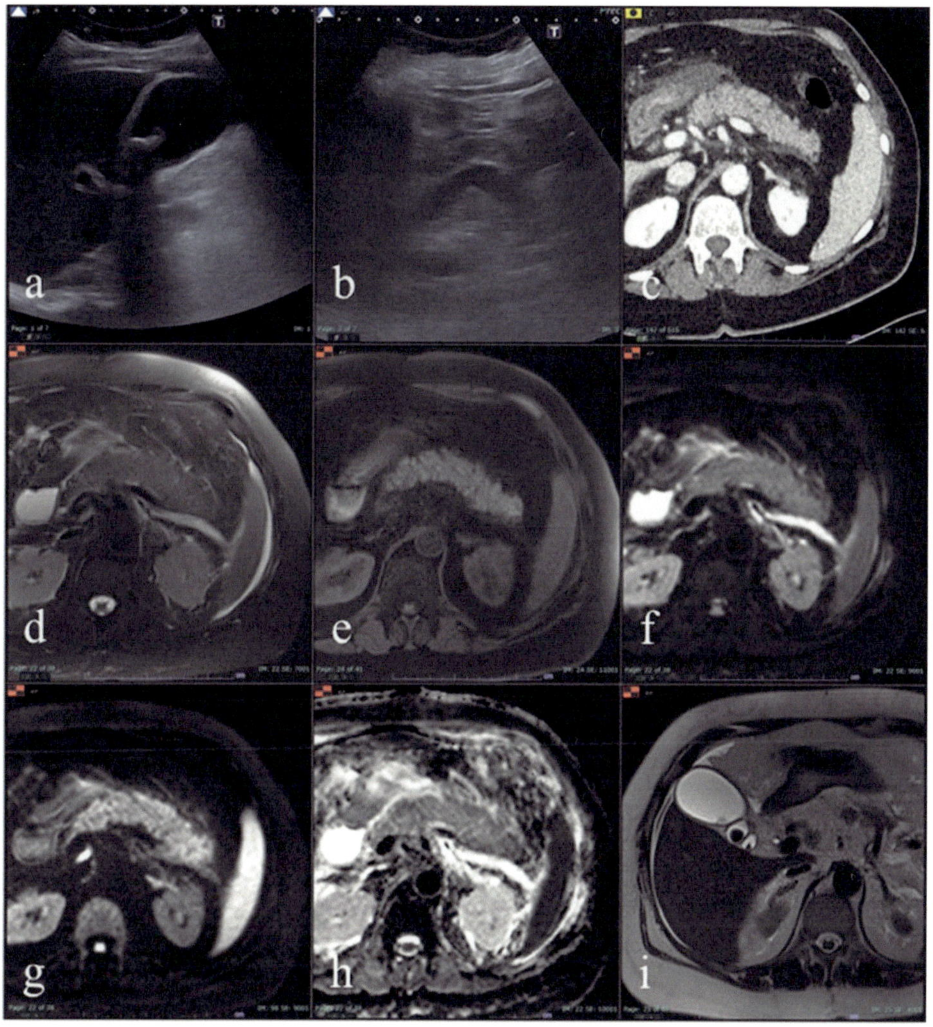

Figure 3.
F, 74 yo with the diagnosis of IEP. Patient with 8x increase of lipase and amylase, pain, gallbladder calculi (a) but a normal-sized pancreas at US (b). At CT (c) no significant alterations of the pancreatic parenchyma are appreciable, but a slight peripancreatic fluid collection in the tail. At MRI, a slight peripancreatic fluid collection is appreciable with different sequences: T2 (d), DWI and ADC map (f, g, h), while pancreatic parenchyma does not show significant alterations at T1WI (e). With DWI, slight parenchymal edema is appreciable in the tail; gallbladder calculi (i).

Criteria distinguishes the collections that contain purely fluid in IEP from the collections that contain also necrotic debris in NP. The distinctions for classifying collections are the time course (≤ 4 or > 4 weeks from the onset of pain) and the presence of necrosis at imaging [1].

APFCs are diagnosed during the first four weeks in patients with IEP; they are peripancreatic homogeneous fluid collections without a wall and tend to conform to the retroperitoneal spaces (**Figure 4**). When a similar collection is seen within the pancreatic parenchyma, it is by definition an ANC and the diagnosis is NP. At MRI APFCs are homogeneously hypointense on T1WI and hyperintense on T2WI [1, 8]. Most APFCs resolve spontaneously, the drainage should not be performed because of

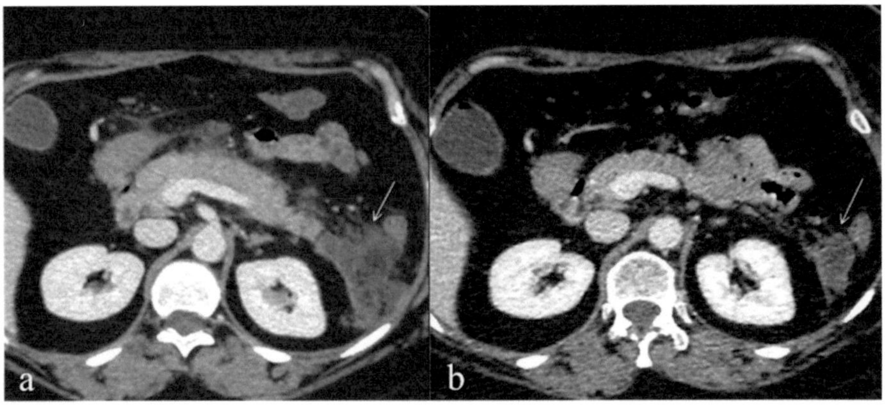

Figure 4.
M, 49 yo. CT images show acute peripancreatic fluid collections (a) within four weeks from the onset of interstitial edematous pancreatitis and the development of a pseudocyst four weeks later (b).

the risk of infecting a sterile collection. Pseudocyst develops in fewer than 10% of IEP when an APFC does not resolve within four weeks and becomes more organized with a wall containing only fluid (**Figure 4**); it is called pseudocyst because lacks a true epithelial tissue. At MRI pseudocysts are uniformly hyperintense on T2WI, with no solid components or debris, and have a thin smooth wall; they may have a connection to the ductal system.

ANCs are poorly organized necrotic collections that develop in NP within the first four weeks of symptoms; they are usually found in the lesser sac, in the pararenal spaces or extended into the pancreatic parenchyma with a lobulated appearance and containing solid or fat debris (**Figure 5**). Any collection associated with an NP should be termed an ANC, even if it is homogeneous without debris. At MRI, ANCs show mixed signals on T1WI and T2WI, with flocculent unenhanced low signal necrotic areas [1, 3, 8]. WON is an ANC that after four weeks develops a thick enhancing wall containing fluid and debris of necrotic fat or pancreatic tissue (**Figure 5**); it may be confined to the pancreatic parenchyma or be in the peripancreatic space. At MRI, a WON shows a well-defined T2-hypointense, gadolinium-enhancing wall and contains non-liquid substances floating [1, 3, 8]. Differentiating a pseudocyst from a WON is important because WON does not respond to endoscopic cyst gastrostomy, but requires surgical debridement [3]. A pseudocyst is peripancreatic with homogeneous

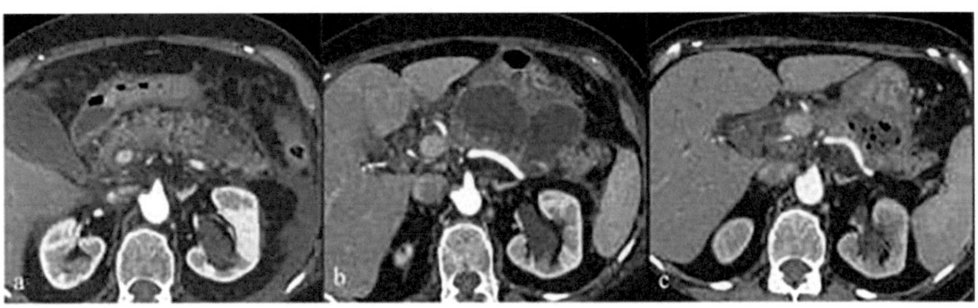

Figure 5.
F, 83 yo. CT follow-up of a patient with necrotizing pancreatitis showing the progression over time from an acute necrotic collection (a) to walled-off necrosis (b); the late infection of the collection (c) required surgical intervention.

DOI: http://dx.doi.org/10.5772/intechopen.106764

fluid, while WON contains necrotic material and can involve both pancreatic and peripancreatic tissue. MRI outperforms CT in the assessment of fluid and necrotic debris in the collections for planning interventions [7].

Any collection can be sterile or infected, the only imaging finding of infection is the presence of gas appearing as multiple small bubbles scattered throughout the collection (**Figure 5**). According to some authors, MRI with DWI shows high sensitivity (100%) and specificity (91%) in detecting infection of collections, even when CT is doubtful due to the lack of bubble gas. On the ADC map the collection shows a target appearance, bright at the center and black at the periphery of the collection, with a similar appearance to a hepatic abscess [9].

The imaging-guided aspiration of fluid collections or the fine-needle aspiration of necrotic tissue can help to diagnose the infection before invasive surgery but can cause iatrogenic infection. Percutaneous drainage is preferred to the fine-needle aspiration because the culture of the fluid can be easily performed; the fine-needle aspiration remains helpful when clinical and imaging findings are confusing [1, 3].

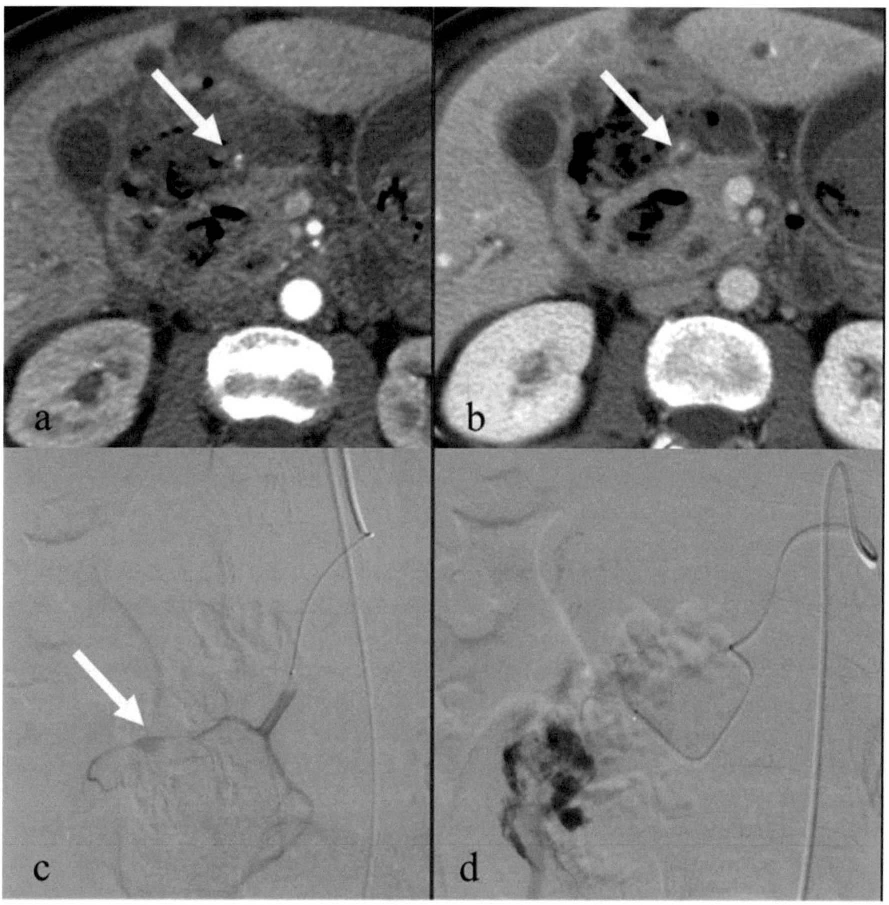

Figure 6.
F, 56 yo with upper gastrointestinal bleeding a month after acute pancreatitis onset; CT detected a pseudoaneurysm of the superior pancreaticoduodenal artery due to walled-off necrosis (a, b). The patient underwent an emergent percutaneous angiography that confirmed the extravasation of the contrast medium (c) and selective embolization of the culprit branches (d).

Pancreatic collections may have an extrapancreatic spread resulting in intrasplenic collection or abscess, splenic infarction or intrasplenic hemorrhage; similar complications may occur in the liver. In these cases, the pancreatic enzymes may extend into the mesenteries and can cause bacterial translocation, bowel ischemia and perforation. Moreover, necrotic collections can erode the bowel wall (especially the wall of the colon and duodenum in 4% of NP) and create a pancreatic-enteric fistula that also manifests gas bubbles in infected collections. Renal involvement is usually due to the inflammatory spread to pararenal spaces, the left space is the one commonly involved by vascular abnormalities [10].

Other main complications are due to the involvement of vascular structures and can lead to developing portal system thrombosis or arterial pseudoaneurysms. Splenic vein thrombosis is the most common complication and may result in gastric varices or splenomegaly [3]. Arterial pseudoaneurysms can lead to life-threatening hemorrhages when the extravasated pancreatic enzymes erode the walls of splenic, pancreaticoduodenal or gastroduodenal arteries [3]. In these cases, the interventional radiology approach is recommended to perform fast and selective vessel embolization with coils or glue (**Figure 6**).

3. Recurrent acute pancreatitis

Recurrent acute pancreatitis (RAP) is a common clinical problem, among the first causes of emergency and expense for gastroenterological pathologies in US [11, 12]. Common complications such as the evolution to episodes of acute pancreatitis, the onset of diabetes or the progression to chronic pancreatitis represent an eventuality with a serious impact on the patient's quality of life and on healthcare costs [13]. About one-third of cases of acute pancreatitis have a recurrence, resulting in the onset of chronic pancreatitis over time [14]. In these cases, it is important since the first episode of pancreatitis to study its causes in order to be able to prevent the onset of new ones, thus avoiding progression to chronic forms. In this sense radiology plays an important role, allowing to identify the causes early and treat them promptly, improving the patient's outcome. In fact, the idiopathic forms of acute pancreatitis, those without an apparent underlying cause that can be treated, have a significantly worse outcome [15].

Clinically it is defined as RAP when two or more episodes of pancreatitis are documented three months apart [14]. The underlying causes of RAP are primarily biliary and alcoholic. There are also rarer causes, such as hypertriglyceridemia, about 5%, autoimmune pancreatitis (AIP) and genetic causes. For this reason, it is always recommended to measure blood triglycerides, search for possible autoimmune etiologies (especially type II AIP), and search for mutations affecting at least four genes, especially in young patients with early onset of acute pancreatitis, in which a genetic mutation exists very frequently [11, 16].

However, radiology is crucial in identifying only some of these causes of recurrent pancreatic inflammation, in particular those of biliary origin, those related to an anomaly of the pancreatic ductal system, a sphincter of Oddi dysfunction (SOD) or other causes of intrapancreatic obstruction.

Although CT and MRI are first-level methods for studying the pancreatic and biliary ductal system, currently the gold standard to identify small calculi or even small tumors that hinder the outflow of pancreatic juice is endoscopic ultrasonography (EUS) [17]. However, this is a highly operator-dependent method, which requires high

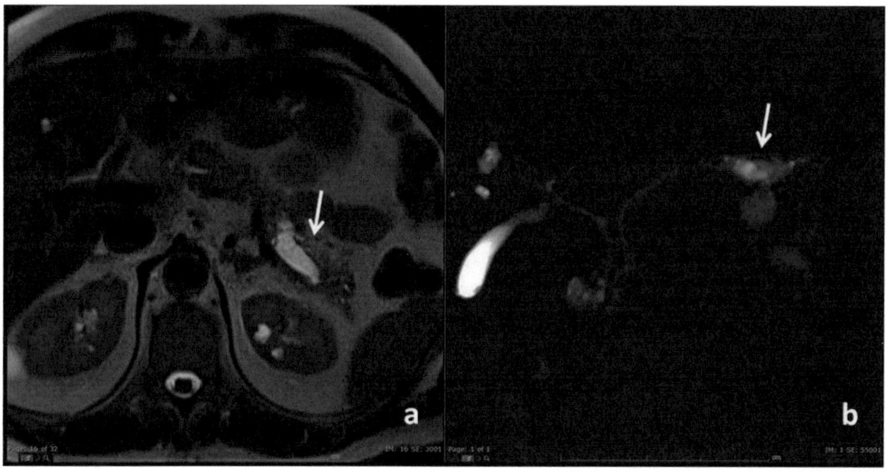

Figure 7.
Male, 66 yo with RAP (3 episodes). Dilatation of the main pancreatic duct (arrows) is appreciable in the tail of the pancreas, both at T2w (a) and MRCP (b), compatible with MD-IPMN.

expertise of the physician and which is not available in all centers. For this reason, CT and MRI are more commonly used. CT is useful for detecting ductal obstructions due to calcific stones. MRI with cholangiopancreatography (MRCP), on the other hand, allows evaluation of the anatomy and possible anomalies of the pancreatic duct and its branches. Both methods allow us to study the pancreatic parenchyma, in order to identify those causes of RAP that originate from parenchymal disease, such as AIP, which will be discussed later. Radiology also has the role of identifying and characterizing any intraductal papillary neoplasms (IPMN), which can be the cause of RAP. Both main duct and branch ducts IPMNs produce mucus, which is viscous and can temporarily obstruct the outflow into the main pancreatic duct, causing small painful colic that can also lead to real episodes of pancreatitis that recur over time. In this case, MRI is essential to characterize pancreatic cystic lesions and above all to clarify their communication with the ductal system in IPMNs (**Figure 7**). Other causes of the obstacle to the outflow of pancreatic juice that can be effectively studied with radiology are congenital variants of pancreatic ducts. The main anatomical anomaly of the ducts is the pancreas divisum (**Figure 8**), in which the pancreatic duct remains divided into its two embryonic components: the ventral duct and the dorsal duct. However, only about 5% of the population has this anatomical variant and among them, only 5% will develop symptoms of RAP [18]. Pancreas divisum is classically classified into three types: type 1 is when there is an incomplete fusion between the ventral and dorsal ducts (more common), type 2 is when there is the total dominance of the dorsal duct with complete absence of the Wirsung duct, while type 3 is when there is a thin communication between the two ducts (incomplete divisum) [19].

MRCP is also important for detecting the presence of a santorinicele with high sensitivity, which can be one of the causes of pancreatic outflow impairment (**Figure 8**).

S-MRCP is a morpho-functional method that requires the administration of secretin to the patient and the serial acquisition of MRCP images to evaluate the various phases of pancreatic secretion in the duodenum [20]. In a healthy pancreas, 1 minute after administration, a filling with minimal dilation of the main pancreatic duct and all the side branches is expected, starting to glimpse a duodenal filling. After 5 minutes the ductal system is completely relaxed and the duodenum filled with liquid. In case

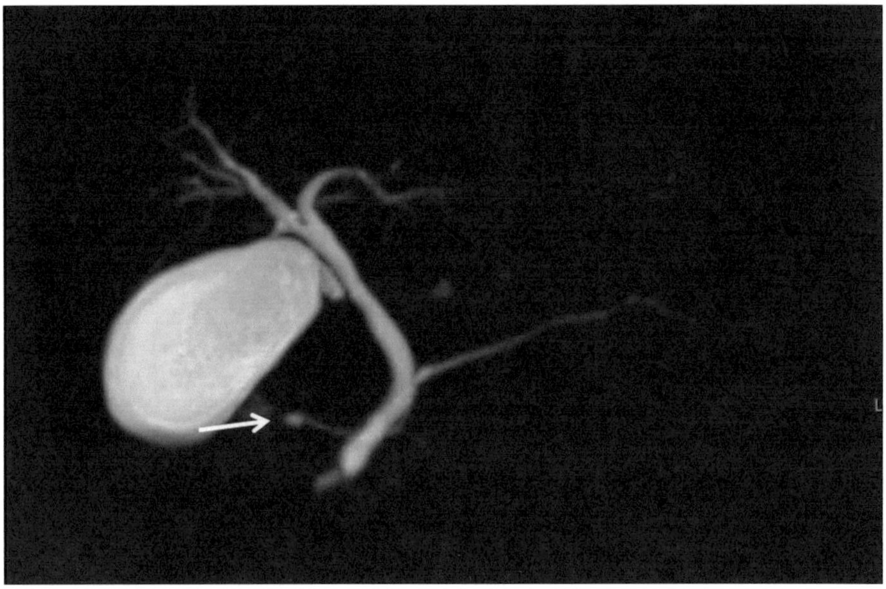

Figure 8.
M, 41 yo. History of recurrent epigastric pain. At MRCP a pancreas divisum is visible with a small ectasia at the level of the minor papilla (santorinicele).

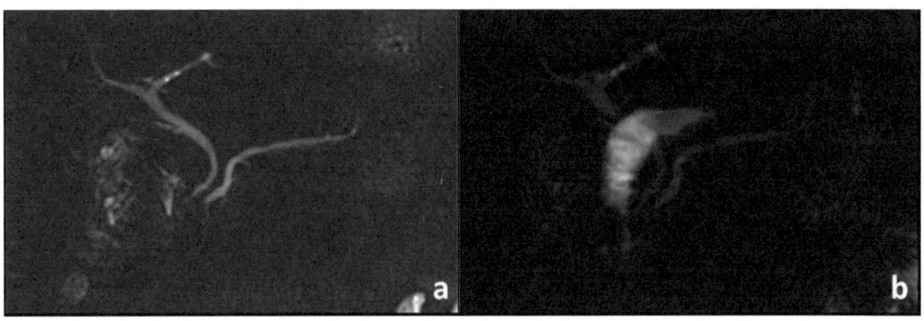

Figure 9.
M, 42 yo. Recurrent abdominal pain with amylase elevation. S-MRCP during (a) and 5 minutes after (b) administration of secretin. The main duct persists dilatated even after 5 minutes, the diagnosis is compatible with SOD. The physiological duodenal filling is delayed but partially conserved.

of impaired functional alterations, such as SOD, which is not detectable with morphological imaging, this physiological flow in the duodenum is not observed and the ductal system remains dilated for a longer time, without emptying regularly (**Figure 9**).

S-MRCP is useful for identifying cases of santorinicele, as well as for evaluating the effects of sphincterotomy [21]. Finally, it is useful for highlighting any anatomical anomalies of the ducts not clearly visible to the common MRCP which can lead to obstructive disease, as previously described.

4. Paraduodenal pancreatitis

Paraduodenal pancreatitis (PDP) is a form of chronic pancreatitis which involves the duodenal wall near the papilla minor and the nearby pancreatic parenchyma or the space interposed between them, named pancreatic groove [22]. The disease is strictly related to ethanol abuse, affecting mainly 40–50 years old males [23]. Clinical manifestations resemble those of chronic pancreatitis, with recurrent pain in the upper abdomen exacerbated by eating, nausea and weight loss. Rarer is obstructive jaundice, which is more typical of pancreatic cancer, but tumor markers are negative [24]. Different pathological entities are grouped in PDP diagnosis. Groove pancreatitis is the most common; it is characterized by the formation of scar tissue between the duodenal wall and the neighbor pancreatic parenchyma, caused by an anatomical or functional obstruction of minor papilla outflow [25, 26]. Even the presence of ectopic pancreatic tissue can cause paraduodenal pancreatitis, leading to paraduodenal wall cysts formation. These usually involve the descending part of the duodenum and are mostly located in the submucosa [24].

In paraduodenal pancreatitis, CT usually shows a hypoattenuating solid mass in the pancreatic groove with duodenal wall thickening often visible, sometimes associated with cystic lesions. The presence of duodenal wall thickening and cystic changes may help to differentiate PDP from pancreatic cancer, where these findings are rare. Duodenal stenosis with gastric outlet obstruction is an uncommon finding but it is more frequent than in pancreatic cancer [27, 28].

MRCP is the gold standard for the study of paraduodenal pancreatic lesions. In solid forms, MRI shows a hypointense lesion near the duodenal wall at T1-weighted imaging, with a variable signal in T2-weighting (**Figure 10**) [29].

The enhancement of these lesions both at CT and MRI is related to their high fibrous content, with a slow progressive enhancement, not visible in the arterial phase, where the lesion appears hypovascular, but with a later homogenous enhancement, thus allowing to distinguish PDP from PDAC, which usually tends to remain hypovascular even in the later acquisition phases (**Figure 10**) [24].

MRI is also fundamental for studying cystic forms of PDP, first of all highlighting their fluid content, and then studying their relationship with the duodenal wall,

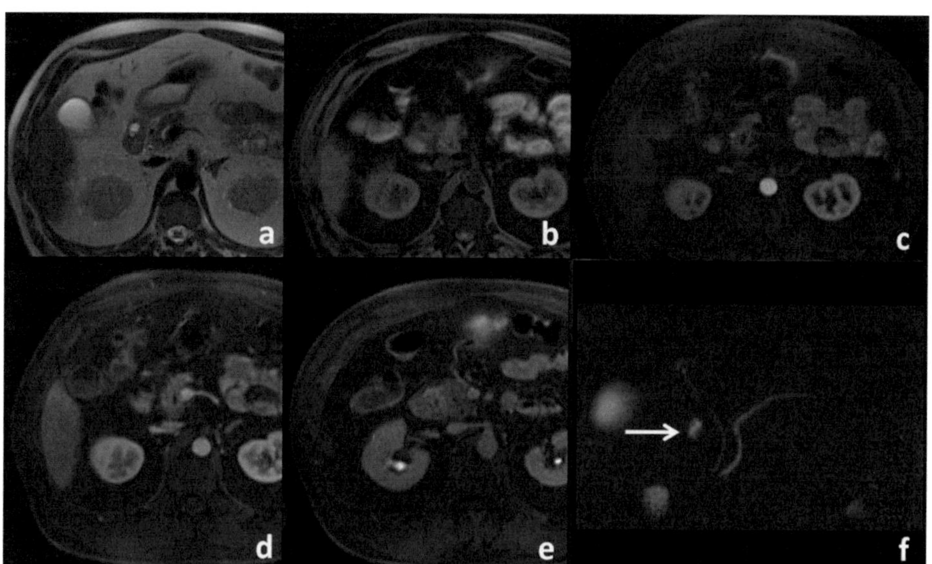

Figure 10.
M, 45 yo. Alcohol abuse. Recurrent epigastric pain. Paraduodenal pancreatitis. A small cystic lesion in the groove area is appreciated (a), embedded in a hypointense soft tissue mass (b), hypovascular (c, d), with delayed enhancement (e). At MRCP the cystic lesion is well appreciated (arrow, f).

with the ductal system and with the healthy pancreatic parenchyma or with fibrotic changes (**Figure 10**). MRCP sequences are essential for evaluating the relationship between the duodenum and intrapancreatic choledochus; in particular, while in pancreatic cancer the choledochus is more frequently irregularly stenotic and infiltrated by the neoplasm, with marked upstream dilation of the biliary tree, in PDP it is more frequently smoothly narrowed and displaced, and therefore the MRCP shows an increase in the physiological space between the choledochus and the lumen of the duodenum (**Figure 10**) [30]. In the same way, the gastroduodenal artery can be displaced in PDP instead of being infiltrated in pancreatic cancer (**Figure 10**).

Although imaging is important for the study of PDP, both for solid and cystic forms, it is not always possible to make a differential diagnosis, in particular with PDAC, cholangiocarcinoma or cancer of the duodenal wall which has a worse prognosis and require different treatments [29, 31]. Laboratory tests and tumor markers can help to sort out the diagnosis, but it is often necessary to combine EUS investigations with tissue sampling to rule out the presence of cancer.

5. Autoimmune pancreatitis

Autoimmune pancreatitis (AIP) is an uncommon form of pancreatitis characterized by frequent the presentation of focal or diffuse pancreatic enlargement with (when the lesion affects the pancreatic head) or without obstructive jaundice, caused by a histological lymphoplasmacytic infiltrate and fibrosis and characterized by a dramatic response to steroids [32]. Two forms of AIP are classified based on clinical and histopathological findings. AIP type 1 is characterized by lymphoplasmacytic sclerosing pancreatitis without granulocyte epithelial lesions, with the presence of dense infiltrate of IgG4 positive plasma cells, being an expression of an IgG4-related systemic disease often characterized by extrapancreatic lesions (i.e., sclerosing cholangitis, sclerosing sialadenitis, and retroperitoneal fibrosis). AIP type 2, on the other hand, refers to idiopathic duct-centric pancreatitis with granulocyte epithelial lesions; this condition does not appear to be associated with IgG4-related systemic disease but it can be associated with an inflammatory bowel disease. In this latter condition, pancreatic enlargement may not be visible but stenosis of the Wirsung duct is characteristic.

The role of radiology in AIP is fundamental, as it can characterize it and distinguish it from PDAC in the case of focal AIP, allowing correct management of this disease.

MRI with MRCP allows both to evaluate the pancreatic parenchyma, its enhancement, and the morphology of the ductal system [33, 34]. Furthermore, DWI imaging, evaluating the microscopic movement of water molecules, can show a restricted diffusion due to the presence of cellular infiltrate that limits the water movement. The imaging findings must be understood considering that histopathology of AIP includes a periductal infiltrate which leads to an increase in the size of the pancreatic gland and at the same time to a compression of the ductal system; another important aspect that characterizes AIP is the presence of obliterating vasculitis [32, 35, 36]. This is important because these two factors, hypovascularization and ductal stenosis, can radiologically mimic pancreatic cancer. Therefore, AIP exhibits imaging features that may be typical or atypical.

Typical AIP is characterized by diffuse ("sausage-like") enlargement of the gland with a loss of physiological lobulation due to an increase in tissue pressure with delayed enhancement, sometimes associated with rim-like enhancement. In AIP at MRCP the main pancreatic duct presents a long reduction of the caliber (more than 1/3 of the length of the main pancreatic duct) or multiple strictures without significant upstream dilatation (**Figure 11**), differently from pancreatic cancer where the stenosis is focal with marked upstream dilatation.

However, some AIP presents with an atypical appearance, showing low-density focal mass at CT, pancreatic duct upstream dilatation, or distal atrophy of the parenchyma. These atypical imaging findings in patients with obstructive jaundice are highly suggestive of pancreatic cancer and should be managed as pancreatic cancer unless there is strong evidence for AIP, and a precise workup for cancer is negative [32]. However, the presence of segmental or focal enlargement of the pancreas with delayed enhancement, highly restricted diffusion and focal narrowing of the main pancreatic duct without marked upstream dilatation (<5 mm), are imaging signs that may aid in the differential diagnosis between atypical AIP and pancreatic cancer

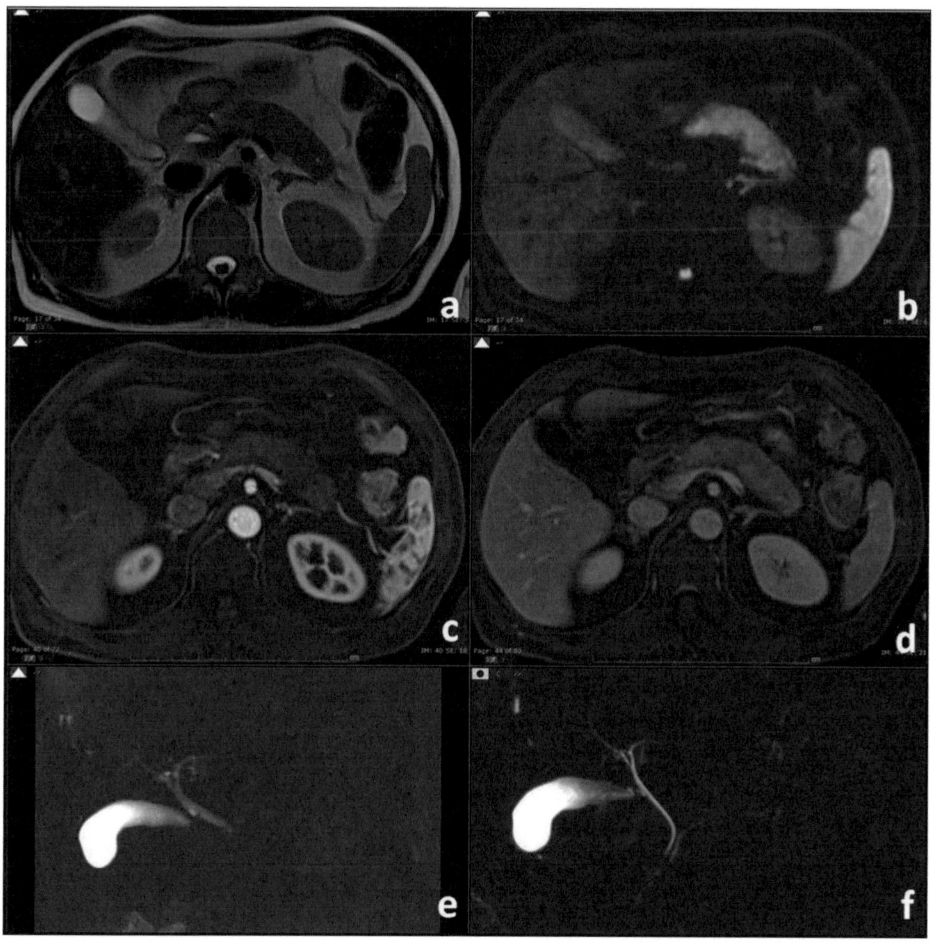

Figure 11.
M, 55 yo. Autoimmune pancreatitis, diffuse form. A diffuse enlargement of the pancreas is appreciable (a), showing restricted diffusion with high signal intensity on DWI (b), hypovascular in the arterial phase (c) but showing late homogeneous enhancement (d). At MRCP (e), the Wirsung duct is not appreciable due to the compression from the enlarged pancreas but returns to normal after steroid therapy (f).

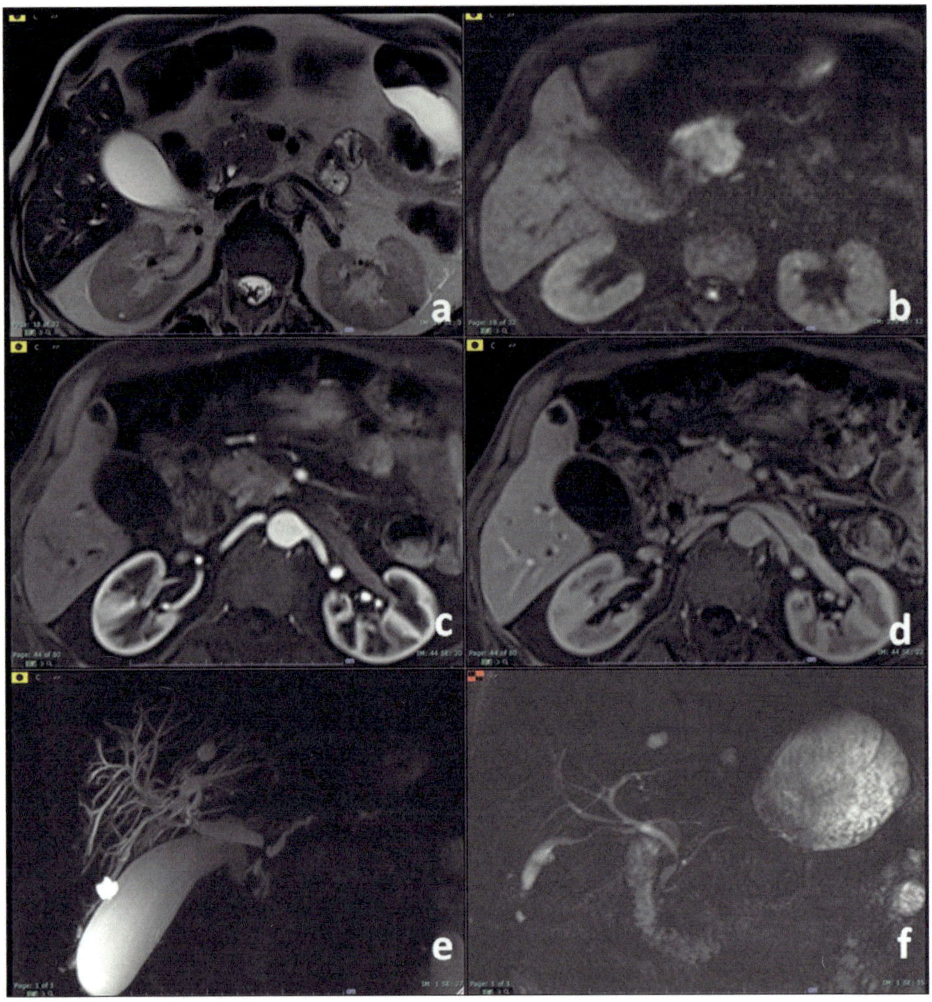

Figure 12.
M, 69 yo. Jaundice. Autoimmune pancreatitis, focal form. A focal enlargement of the head of the pancreas is appreciable (a), showing restricted diffusion with high signal intensity on DWI (b), hypovascular in the arterial phase (c) but showing late homogeneous enhancement (d). At MRCP (e), marked stenosis both of the Wirsung duct and choledochus is appreciable, simulating a "double duct sign", typical of PDAC. After steroid therapy (f) both Wirsung duct and choledochus return to normal.

(**Figure 12**). If the stenosis is focal and single, the possibility of pancreatic cancer is high, but if the stenosis is two or more, it could be a case of atypical AIP [37, 38].

6. Chronic pancreatitis

Chronic pancreatitis (CP) is a pathologic fibroinflammatory syndrome of the pancreas in individuals with genetic, environmental and/or other risk factors who develop persistent pathologic response to parenchymal injury or stress.

CP is most commonly caused by toxins such as alcohol or tobacco, genetic polymorphisms and recurrent attacks of acute pancreatitis.

Early diagnosis of CP is fundamental because early CP is the stage in which target therapy is likely to be most effective.

According to American College of Gastroenterology 2020 guidelines, in patients with clinical symptoms of a pancreatic inflammatory disorder and/or in patients with a suggestive gene–environment risk assessment, cross-sectional imaging, in particular, CT or MRI with MRCP, should be the first-line tests for the diagnosis of CP, because they are valid, reproducible, widely available and non-invasive. Because of its invasiveness and minor reproducibility and availability, EUS should be used after cross-sectional imaging when the diagnosis is still in doubt, or if there is a concern about "minimal changes" that cannot be visualized on cross-sectional imaging. If CT, MRI with MRCP and EUS do not confirm the diagnosis of CP and the suspicion is still high, S-MRCP is suggested because it allows better visualization of the main pancreatic duct and side branches and allows to obtain a semiquantitative measurement of duodenal filling [39].

In CP impaired outflow of pancreatic juice induces inflammation and fibrotic replacement of pancreatic parenchyma; fibrosis is responsible for reduced ductal compliance and ductal anomalies (such as side branches ectasia in early-stage and dilatations, strictures and irregularities of the main pancreatic duct in advances stages), while inflammation causes intraductal and parenchymal calcifications.

At imaging, in early chronic pancreatitis morphology and dimensions of the pancreas are normal, but impairment of pancreatic juice outflow drives mild fibrosis; in overt CP, the main pancreatic duct is dilatated and distorted, pancreatic parenchyma is thinned and may contain cysts, and intraductal and parenchymal calcifications are present.

The role of the radiologist in the early stage is to make a diagnosis of CP and look for its causes (so that they can be removed if possible), while in the advanced phase the role of the radiologist is to confirm the diagnosis, look for its causes, identify complications, monitor the disease and early detect pancreatic adenocarcinoma (PDAC) for which these patients are at increased risk [40]. The most valid radiological techniques to diagnose and monitor CP are CT, MRI with MRCP and S-MRCP.

CT and MRI have similar sensitivity and specificity in diagnosing CP, respectively 75% and 91% for CT and 78% and 98% for MRI [41]. CT is cheaper, easily available, allows rapid visualization and characterization of calcifications and is much faster, thus can be used also in uncooperative patients; on the other hand, MRI allows better identification of early parenchymal alteration and subtle ductal changes so it is the best technique to diagnose early CP; moreover, it is the best technique to monitor disease progression, to early detect pancreatic ductal adenocarcinoma (for which patients with CP are at increased risk) and is useful in differentiating focal CP from PDAC and CP from IPMN. In any case, the two techniques may be considered complementary.

6.1 MRI imaging

MRI is the best technique to early diagnose and follow up CP, thanks to its intrinsic high contrast resolution because it provides optimal visualization of the pancreatic ductal system.

MRCP are key sequences for evaluating the pancreatic ductal system and are acquired using 2D and/or 3D heavily T2 weighted sequences in which structures containing static fluid appear markedly hyperintense while surrounding solid structures display very low signal and appear markedly hypointense (**Figures 8–12**).

The best sequence to evaluate pancreatic borders and pancreatic parenchyma is GRE T1 fat-sat (either with Dixon technique), because of the intrinsic signal differences between the high signal intensity of the pancreatic parenchyma and the suppressed signal of the peri-pancreatic fat. With this sequence, the healthy pancreas, whose cells are rich in proteins, appears homogeneously hyperintense while the fibrotic replacement of acinar cells leads to a progressive decrease in signal intensity, and this signal loss correlates with the decrease in exocrine function (**Figures 13** and **14**) [42, 43].

Moreover with "T1 mapping", a novel advanced MRI technique, pancreatic T1 signal intensity may be reliably assessed and could be used as a practical and sensitive biomarker to monitor CP and to diagnose mild CP, even earlier than ductal anomalies become appreciable, as the fibrotic replacement of acinar cells precedes ductal alterations (**Figure 15**). T1 mapping is a quantitative MR imaging technique that allows measuring the tissue-specific T1 relaxation time. The T1 relaxation time of pancreatic parenchyma is significantly increased in patients with mild CP [44] and, given the quantitative nature of the data, T1 mapping may be a more reliable method compared to traditional T1 weighted imaging, allowing ready comparison across longitudinal time points and permitting a more meaningful interpretation of intensity changes, so it could become a biomarker. However, more studies are required to transform these potential benefits into clinical practice.

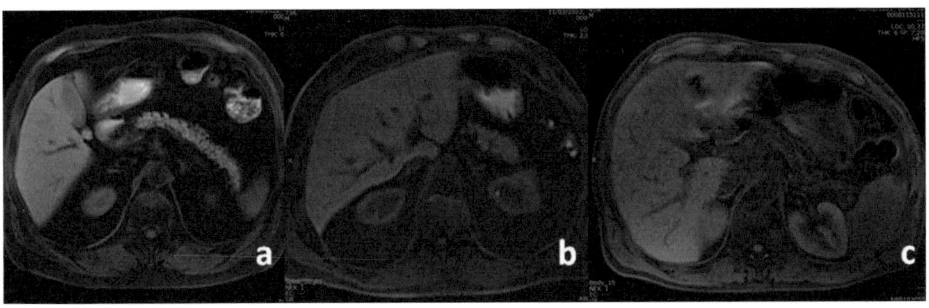

Figure 13.
T1w GRE fat-sat MRI scan comparing a normal pancreas (a), a mild CP (b) and an advanced CP (c), where the non-enhanced T1 intensity of the gland is gradually reduced according to the severity of CP.

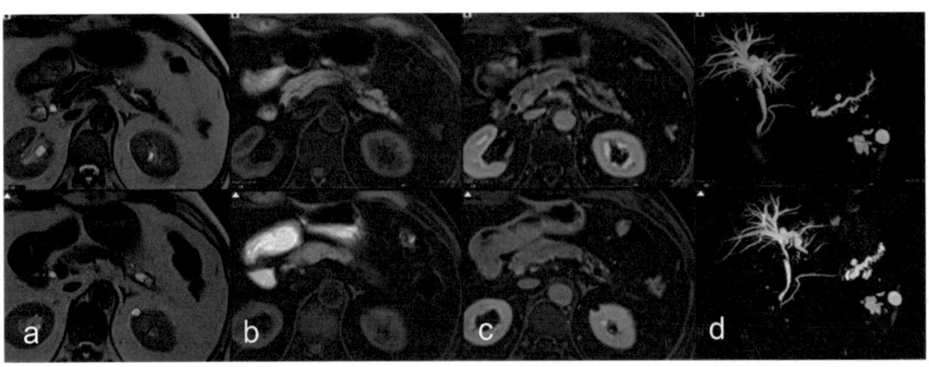

Figure 14.
M, 70 yo. Evolution of CP few months (up) and few years (down) after necrotizing pancreatitis recovery in T2w HASTE sequence (a), unenhanced T1w GRE fat-sat (b), delayed-phase T1w GRE fat-sat (c) and MRCP (d). The progressive upstream dilatation of the ductal system is accompanied by a progressive reduction of T1 intensity of the parenchyma which is increasingly replaced by fibrosis.

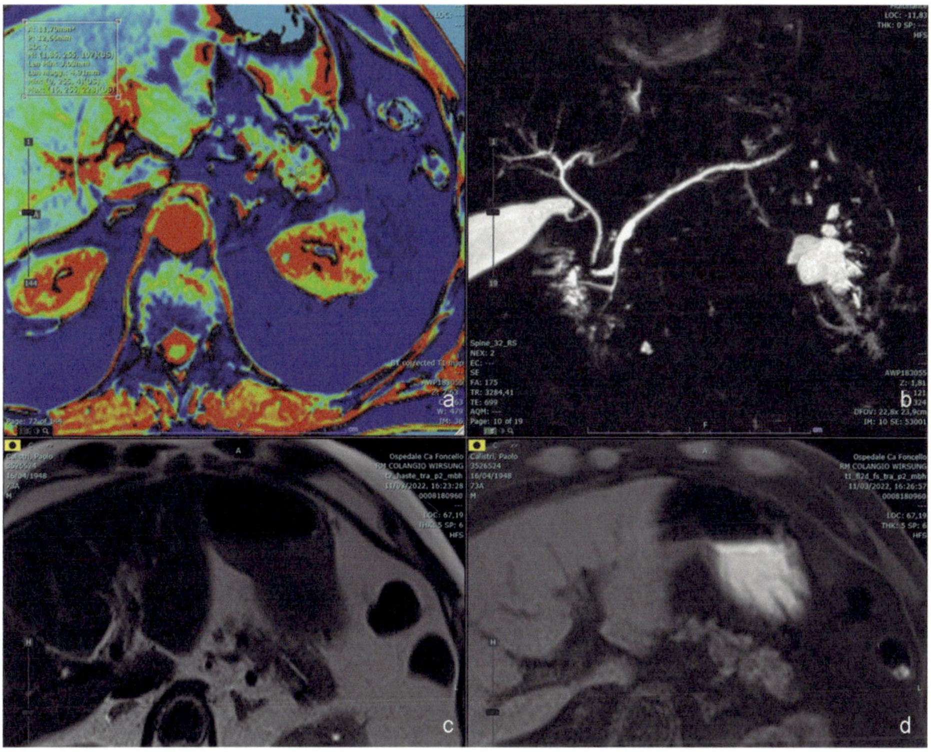

Figure 15.
M, 73 yo. Early-stage of CP in T1 mapping sequence (a), S-MRCP (b), T2w HASTE sequence c), unenhanced T1w GRE fat-sat (d). T1-mapping shows an increased T1 relaxation time of the gland even before the appearance of marked classic signs of chronic pancreatitis. S-MRCP visualization of side branches at body-tail after secretin is a sign of early CP.

After contrast injection, while a healthy pancreas typically displays strong enhancement in the arterial phase and homogeneously decreasing enhancement in the venous phase, in CP fibrotic tissue causes heterogeneously reduced enhancement in the arterial phase, followed by a delayed enhancement in the venous and equilibrium phase, related to the fibrotic changes of the pancreatic parenchyma (**Figure 14**) [28, 43].

The ductal abnormalities are well depicted on MRCP images. In particular, in the early-stage CP side branches get mildly dilatated and become visible, while in advanced stages are depicted more severe alterations of side branches (such as ectasia or sacculation) and alterations of the main duct such as irregular profiles, dilatation, focal strictures and filling defects (due to stones and protein plugs). Ductal abnormalities of CP can be scored according to the Cambridge Classification modified for MRCP (**Table 2**) [45].

The overall sensitivity of MRCP for diagnosing CP increases from 77–89% using S-MRCP [46], which adds both morphological and functional information. Secretin infusion induces transitory hypertension in the ductal system improving the morphological evaluation of the main pancreatic duct and side branches and making eventual ducts anatomical variants (such as pancreas divisum), obstructions, stenosis, dilatations and irregular contours easier detectable.

In a healthy pancreas, ductal response to secretin stimulation determines an increase in the main duct caliber of approximately 1 mm with a peak at 3 min with

Grading	Imaging findings
I (normal pancreas)	Pancreatic ducts are normal
II (equivocal pancreas)	1–2 side branches and main duct 2–4 mm
III (mild disease)	≥ 3 side branches and main duct 2–4 mm
IV (moderate disease)	≥ 3 side branches and main duct >4 mm
V (marked disease)	As above with one or more among large cavities (10 mm), gland enlargement (>2x), intraductal filling defects or calculi, duct obstruction, gross irregularity or contiguous organ invasion

Table 2.
Grading of chronic pancreatitis.

the return to baseline caliber at 10 min. In CP periductal fibrosis causes a decrease in ductal compliance and leads to an abnormal and persistent main duct dilatation with visibility of the side branches. Thus, visualization of side branches at the body-tail after secretin is a sign of early CP (**Figure 15**) [47]. Moreover, in early stages of CP, secretin-induced hypertension may result in acinar filling with a progressive hydrographic enhancement of the pancreatic parenchyma, the so-called "S-MRCP parenchymogram" which is a sign of pancreatic outlet obstruction (**Figure 16**) [43, 48].

Finally, S-MRCP allows to obtain a semiquantitative assessment of the duodenal filling which correlates with pancreatic exocrine function, with diagnostic performance comparable to that of invasive tests such as endoscopic pancreatic function testing [49]. The semiquantitative assessment is performed by applying a grading system to duodenal filling from grade I (filling limited to the duodenal bulb, indicating severely reduced duodenal filling), to grade II (filling visible as far as the second portion of the duodenum, indicating reduced duodenal filling),

to grade III (filling beyond the second portion of the duodenum, indicating normal duodenal filling); a reduced duodenal filling suggests a decrease in pancreatic exocrine reserve. However, the normal duodenal filling does not exclude impairment of pancreatic exocrine function; so reduced duodenal filling is a specific but not sensitive sign of CP.

In some cases, CP can be focal and thus simulates PDAC and differential diagnosis is very difficult, even for the pathologist, because PDAC is characterized by a rich desmoplastic component.

To make a correct diagnosis, the radiologist can rely both on morphological criteria (in the particular relationship between the lesion and the dilatated ducts, the

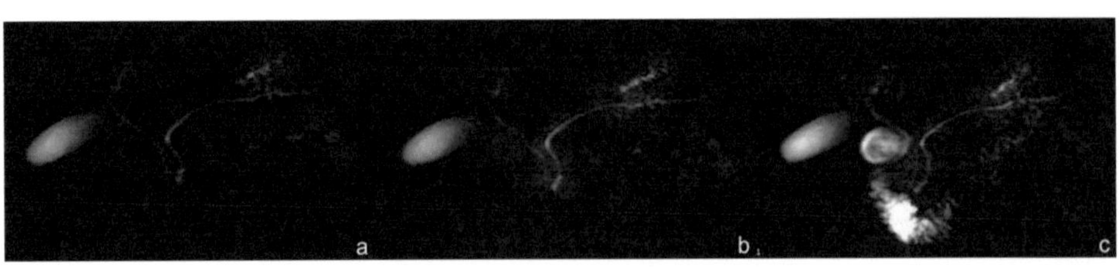

Figure 16.
M, 45 yo, Recurrent episodes of pain and increase of pancreatic enzymes. Pre-secretin MRCP (a) shows no significant changes. Just 2 minutes after secretin injection (b), an increase in signal intensity of the parenchyma can be observed and persists for the full 17 minutes of the exam (c). This phase shows a good passage of pancreatic juice in the duodenum due to adequate exocrine function.

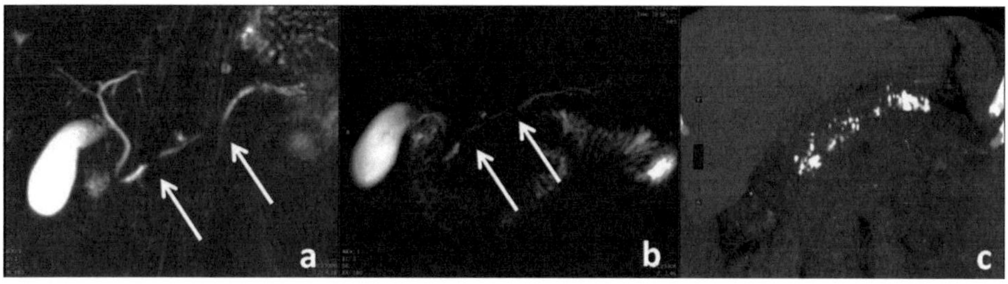

Figure 17.
M, 65 yo. CP with evidence of two ductal strictures at MRCP sequences (arrows) at diagnosis (a) and a few months later (b). CT (c) performed two years later discovers multiple gross calcifications of pancreatic parenchyma, typical of CP.

relationship between the lesion and calcifications and enhancement criteria) and on functional criteria (in particularly advanced DWI techniques and S-MRCP).

In PDAC both pancreatic dilatated ducts and calcifications are displaced at the periphery of the lesion, while in focal CP calcification and dilatated ducts are part of the lesion and so are located within it.

Both focal CP and PDAC are hypointense in T1 fat-sat and hypovascular in the pancreatic arterial phase, but while PDAC most of the time persists hypovascular, in focal CP a delayed enhancement is often detected.

Both focal CP and PDAC cause stenosis of the main duct, however, while in focal CP the stenoses reduce or resolve after secretin stimulation (duct penetrating sign), it does not change in PDAC (**Figure 17**) [50].

As the risk of pancreatic cancer is significantly elevated in patients with CP (cumulative risk at 10 and 20 years after the diagnosis of pancreatitis, respectively 1.8 and 4% [40]), this population needs to be followed up also to early detect PDAC, when the lesion is still resectable. MRI with MRCP and eventually with s MRCP is the best technique to early detect PDAC since very often the first sign of PDAC onset is focal stenosis of the main duct that does not resolve after secretin stimulation.

In advanced CP, the aspect of the pancreatic ductal system may mimic that of the main duct intraductal papillary mucinous neoplasm (MD-IPMN); however in MD-IPMN the dilatation of the main duct is more homogeneous with regular margins and without strictures, usually associated with bulging ampulla, sometimes with grape-like secondary duct dilatation and with a solid nodule in a duct, while specific findings of CP are ductal dilatation with strictures, the presence of a stone and side branches ectasia with non-cystic appearance (**Figure 18**) [51].

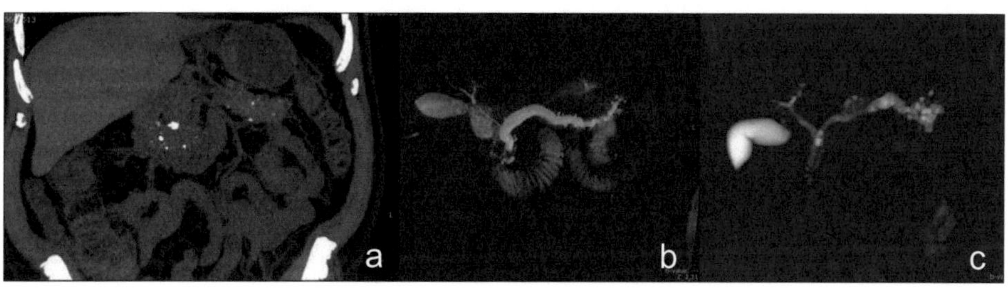

Figure 18.
CP with multiple calcifications at CT scan (a) and diffuse dilatation of ductal system at MRCP (b), compared to a mixed IPMN with main duct IPMN component clearly visible at MRCP (c).

In conclusion, nowadays MRI is the best technique to early detect and monitor CP, to early detect PDAC in patients with CP and make a differential diagnosis between PDAC and focal CP and between MD-IPMN and CP. In the future MRI with T1 mapping could provide a biomarker to detect and monitor CP [52].

6.2 CT imaging

CT has been a cornerstone for evaluating CP, thanks to its availability and reliability. Even if MRI has superior accuracy for imaging the ductal system, CT with its high spatial can well depict both the parenchyma and the dilatated ducts in a few minutes and provides good-quality morphological information even in uncooperative patients; moreover, CT is the best technique to detect and study the structure of parenchymal and intraductal calcifications, and to identify CP complications such as pseudocysts, vascular thrombosis and pseudoaneurysm [52].

Unenhanced CT may be considered complementary to MRI and MRCP because it allows to easily identify and precisely localize both pancreatic parenchymal and ductal calcifications (important information for treatment planning) (**Figure 19**), and permits to study the structure of stones, in order to identify features suggestive of gene mutations associated with CP. In particular stones with a hypodense central core, with the so-called "bull's eye" appearance, are detected in 67% of patients with a gene mutation associated CP [53] and identifying these patients is important because they have an even higher risk of developing PDAC and thus require strict surveillance, genetic counseling and family testing.

During the pancreatic parenchymal phase (a late arterial phase acquired approximately 40 s after the initiation of intravenous contrast injection) parenchymal enhancement is typically reduced in CP, due to fibrotic changes. Moreover, complications such as fluid collection and vascular abnormalities like pseudoaneurysms are detected. In the portal venous phase (70–90 s after intravenous contrast medium injection) venous vessels can be adequately studied and complications such as fluid collection and vascular abnormalities like thrombosis are detected [43].

Although CT represents a reliable technique to study patients with CP, it has some important limits. First of all, CT has low sensitivity to detect minimal pancreatic and ductal changes, thus a negative CT does not rule out an early/mild CP [54]. Moreover, CT causes patient exposure to ionizing radiations, which raises concerns for longitudinal monitoring in particular for younger patients, and finally it has rather low

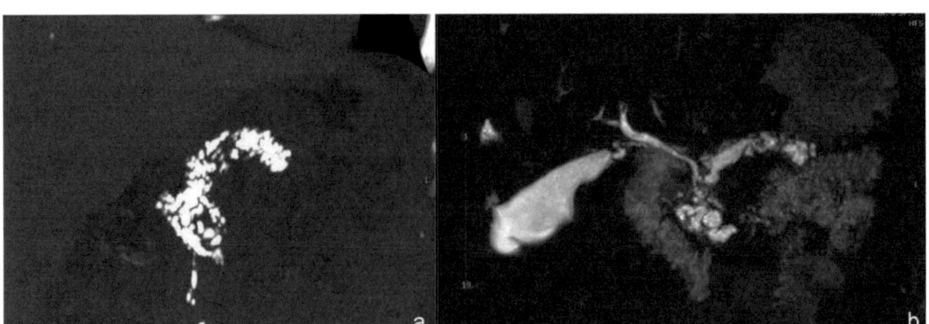

Figure 19.
M, 48 yo. Chronic calcific pancreatitis with multiple gross calcifications in the dilatated ductal system (a), invisible at MRCP sequence (b).

sensitivity (58–77%) to detect small iso-attenuating PDAC because of its non-optimal contrast resolution [55, 56].

7. Conclusion

Imaging of pancreatitis is complex. CT and MRI, also flanked by modern S-MRCP techniques and in the future by T1-mapping, allow their early differential diagnosis, the search for the underlying causes, guide the therapeutic path and the response to therapy, allowing careful follow-up.

Author details

Giovanni Morana*, Alessandro Beleù, Francesca Nistri and Silvia Venturini
Radiological Department, General Hospital "Ca Foncello", Treviso, Italy

*Address all correspondence to: giovanni.morana@aulss2.veneto.it

References

[1] Foster BR, Jensen KK, Bakis G, Shaaban AM, Coakley FV. Revised Atlanta classification for acute pancreatitis: A pictorial essay. Radiology. 2016;**36**:675-687

[2] Colvin SD, Smith EN, Morgan DE, Porter KK. Acute pancreatitis: An update on the revised Atlanta classification. Abdominal Radiology. 2020;**45**:1222-1231

[3] Shyu JY, Sainani NI, Sahni VA, Chick JF, Chauhan NR, Conwell DL, et al. Necrotizing pancreatitis: Diagnosis, imaging, and intervention. Radiology. 2014;**34**:1218-1239

[4] Tenner S, Baillie J, DeWitt J, Vege SS. American College of Gastroenterology guideline: Management of acute pancreatitis. American Journal of Gastroenterology. 2013;**108**:1400-1415 1416

[5] Zhao K, Adam SZ, Keswani RN, Horowitz JM, Miller FH. Acute pancreatitis: Revised Atlanta classification and the role of cross-sectional imaging. AJR American Journal of Roentgenology. 2015;**205**:W32-W41

[6] Thoeni RF. The revised Atlanta classification of acute pancreatitis: Its importance for the radiologist and its effect on treatment. Radiology. 2012;**262**:751-764

[7] Morgan DE, Baron TH, Smith JK, Robbin ML, Kenney PJ. Pancreatic fluid collections prior to intervention: Evaluation with MR imaging compared with CT and US. Radiology. 1997;**203**:773-778

[8] Sun H, Zuo H-D, Lin Q, Yang D-D, Zhou T, Tang M-Y, et al. MR imaging for acute pancreatitis: The current status of clinical applications. Annals of Translational Medicine. 2019;**7**:269

[9] Islim F, Salik AE, Bayramoglu S, Guven K, Alis H, Turhan AN. Non-invasive detection of infection in acute pancreatic and acute necrotic collections with diffusion-weighted magnetic resonance imaging: Preliminary findings. Abdominal Imaging. 2014;**39**:472-481

[10] Mortelé KJ, Mergo PJ, Taylor HM, Wiesner W, Cantisani V, Ernst MD, et al. Peripancreatic vascular abnormalities complicating acute pancreatitis: Contrast-enhanced helical CT findings. European Journal of Radiology. 2004;**52**:67-72

[11] Guda NM, Muddana V, Whitcomb DC, Levy P, Garg P, Cote G, et al. Recurrent acute pancreatitis: International state-of-the-science conference with recommendations. Pancreas. 2018;**47**:653-666

[12] Peery AF, Crockett SD, Murphy CC, Lund JL, Dellon ES, Williams JL, et al. Burden and cost of gastrointestinal, liver, and pancreatic diseases in the United States: Update 2018. Gastroenterology. 2019;**156**:254-272.e11

[13] Mathews SC, Izmailyan S, Brito FA, Yamal J-M, Mikhail O, Revere FL. Prevalence and financial burden of digestive diseases in a commercially insured population. Clinical Gastroenterology. 2022;**20**(7):1480-1487.e7

[14] Whitcomb DC, Frulloni L, Garg P, Greer JB, Schneider A, Yadav D, et al. Chronic pancreatitis: An international draft consensus proposal for a new mechanistic definition. Pancreatology Official Journal. 2016;**16**:218-224

[15] Poddar U, Yachha SK, Borkar V, Srivastava A. Is acute recurrent pancreatitis in children a precursor of chronic pancreatitis? A long-term follow-up study of 93 cases. Digestive Liver Diseases. 2017;**49**:796-801

[16] IAP/APA evidence-based guidelines for the management of acute pancreatitis. Pancreatology Official Journal. 2013;**13**:e1-e15

[17] Wan J, Ouyang Y, Yu C, Yang X, Xia L, Lu N. Comparison of EUS with MRCP in idiopathic acute pancreatitis: A systematic review and meta-analysis. Gastrointestinal Endoscocpy. 2018;**87**:1180-1188.e9

[18] Ferri V, Vicente E, Quijano Y, Ielpo B, Duran H, Diaz E, et al. Diagnosis and treatment of pancreas divisum: A literature review. Hepatobiliary Pancreat Diseases. 2019;**18**:332-336

[19] Türkvatan A, Erden A, Türkoğlu MA, Yener Ö. Congenital variants and anomalies of the pancreas and pancreatic duct: Imaging by magnetic resonance cholangiopancreaticography and multidetector computed tomography. Korean Journal of Radiology. 2013;**14**:905-913

[20] Matos C, Metens T, Devière J, Nicaise N, Braudé P, Van Yperen G, et al. Pancreatic duct: Morphologic and functional evaluation with dynamic MR pancreatography after secretin stimulation. Radiology. 1997;**203**:435-441

[21] Boninsegna E, Manfredi R, Ventriglia A, Negrelli R, Pedrinolla B, Mehrabi S, et al. Santorinicele: Secretin-enhanced magnetic resonance cholangiopancreatography findings before and after minor papilla sphincterotomy. European Journal of Radiology. 2015;**25**:2437-2444

[22] Adsay NV, Zamboni G. Paraduodenal pancreatitis: A clinico-pathologically distinct entity unifying "cystic dystrophy of heterotopic pancreas", "Para-duodenal wall cyst", and "groove pancreatitis". Seminars in Diagnosed Pathology. 2004;**21**:247-254

[23] Stevens T, Conwell DL, Zuccaro G. Pathogenesis of chronic pancreatitis: An evidence-based review of past theories and recent developments. American Journal of Gastroenterology. 2004;**99**:2256-2270

[24] Arora A, Dev A, Mukund A, Patidar Y, Bhatia V, Sarin SK. Paraduodenal pancreatitis. Clinical Radioloy. 2014;**69**:299-306

[25] Becker V, Mischke U. Groove pancreatitis. International Journal of Pancreatology. 1991;**10**:173-182

[26] Shudo R, Obara T, Tanno S, Fujii T, Nishino N, Sagawa M, et al. Segmental groove pancreatitis accompanied by protein plugs in Santorini's duct. Journal of Gastroenterology. 1998;**33**:289-294

[27] Procacci C, Graziani R, Zamboni G, Cavallini G, Pederzoli P, Guarise A, et al. Cystic dystrophy of the duodenal wall: Radiologic findings. Radiology. 1997;**205**:741-747

[28] Perez-Johnston R, Sainani NI, Sahani DV. Imaging of chronic pancreatitis (including groove and autoimmune pancreatitis). Radiology Clinical North America. 2012;**50**:447-466

[29] Blasbalg R, Baroni RH, Costa DN, Machado MCC. MRI features of groove pancreatitis. AJR American Journal of Roentgenology. 2007;**189**:73-80

[30] Hernandez-Jover D, Pernas JC, Gonzalez-Ceballos S, Lupu I, Monill JM, Pérez C. Pancreatoduodenal junction:

Review of anatomy and pathologic conditions. Journal of Gastrointestinal Surgery. 2011;**15**:1269-1281

[31] Triantopoulou C, Dervenis C, Giannakou N, Papailiou J, Prassopoulos P. Groove pancreatitis: A diagnostic challenge. European Journal of Radiology. 2009;**19**:1736-1743

[32] Shimosegawa T, Chari ST, Frulloni L, Kamisawa T, Kawa S, Mino-Kenudson M, et al. International consensus diagnostic criteria for autoimmune pancreatitis: Guidelines of the International Association of Pancreatology. Pancreas. 2011;**40**:352-358

[33] Wallner BK, Schumacher KA, Weidenmaier W, Friedrich JM. Dilated biliary tract: Evaluation with MR cholangiography with a T2-weighted contrast-enhanced fast sequence. Radiology. 1991;**181**:805-808

[34] Morimoto K, Shimoi M, Shirakawa T, Aoki Y, Choi S, Miyata Y, et al. Biliary obstruction: Evaluation with three-dimensional MR cholangiography. Radiology. 1992;**183**:578-580

[35] Zamboni G, Lüttges J, Capelli P, Frulloni L, Cavallini G, Pederzoli P, et al. Histopathological features of diagnostic and clinical relevance in autoimmune pancreatitis: A study on 53 resection specimens and 9 biopsy specimens. Virchows Archives in Germany. 2004;**445**:552-563

[36] Klöppel G, Sipos B, Zamboni G, Kojima M, Morohoshi T. Autoimmune pancreatitis: Histo- and immunopathological features. Journal of Gastroenterology. 2007;**42** (Suppl. 1):28-31

[37] Negrelli R, Boninsegna E, Avesani G, Zamboni GA, Brozzi L, Frulloni L, et al. Type 1 and type 2 autoimmune pancreatitis: Distinctive clinical and pathological features, but are there any differences at magnetic resonance? Experience from a referral Center. Pancreas. 2018;**47**:1115-1122

[38] Manfredi R, Graziani R, Cicero C, Frulloni L, Carbognin G, Mantovani W, et al. Autoimmune pancreatitis: CT patterns and their changes after steroid treatment. Radiology. 2008;**247**:435-443

[39] Gardner TB, Adler DG, Forsmark CE, Sauer BG, Taylor JR, Whitcomb DC. ACG clinical guideline: Chronic pancreatitis. Americaan Journal of Gastroenterology. 2020;**115**:322-339

[40] Lowenfels AB, Maisonneuve P, Cavallini G, Ammann RW, Lankisch PG, Andersen JR, et al. Pancreatitis and the risk of pancreatic cancer. New England Journal of Medicine. 1993;**328**:1433-1437

[41] Beyer G, Habtezion A, Werner J, Lerch MM, Mayerle J. Chronic pancreatitis. Lancet. 2020;**396**:499-512

[42] Tirkes T, Fogel EL, Sherman S, Lin C, Swensson J, Akisik F, et al. Detection of exocrine dysfunction by MRI in patients with early chronic pancreatitis. Abdominal Radiology (New York). 2017;**42**:544-551

[43] Zamboni GA, Ambrosetti MC, Pezzullo M, Bali MA, Mansueto G. Optimum imaging of chronic pancreatitis. Abdominal Radiology. 2020;**45**: 1410-1419

[44] Tirkes T, Lin C, Fogel EL, Sherman SS, Wang Q, Sandrasegaran K. T(1) mapping for diagnosis of mild chronic pancreatitis. Journal of Magnetic Resonance Imaging. 2017;**45**:1171-1176

[45] Hansen TM, Nilsson M, Gram M, Frøkjær JB. Morphological and functional evaluation of

chronic pancreatitis with magnetic resonance imaging. World Journal of Gastroenterology. 2013;**19**:7241-7246

[46] Hellerhoff KJ, Helmberger H 3rd, Rösch T, Settles MR, Link TM, Rummeny EJ. Dynamic MR pancreatography after secretin administration: Image quality and diagnostic accuracy. AJR American Journal of Roentgenology. 2002;**179**:121-129

[47] Tirkes T, Sandrasegaran K, Sanyal R, Sherman S, Schmidt CM, Cote GA, et al. Secretin-enhanced MR cholangiopancreatography: Spectrum of findings. Radiology. 2013;**33**:1889-1906

[48] Matos C, Devière J, Cremer M, Nicaise N, Struyven J, Metens T. Acinar filling during secretin-stimulated MR pancreatography. AJR American Journal of Roentgenology. 1998;**171**:165-169

[49] Cappeliez O, Delhaye M, Devière J, Le Moine O, Metens T, Nicaise N, et al. Chronic pancreatitis: Evaluation of pancreatic exocrine function with MR pancreatography after secretin stimulation. Radiology. 2000;**215**:358-364

[50] Ichikawa T, Sou H, Araki T, Arbab AS, Yoshikawa T, Ishigame K, et al. Duct-penetrating sign at MRCP: Usefulness for differentiating inflammatory pancreatic mass from pancreatic carcinomas. Radiology. 2001;**221**:107-116

[51] Kim JH, Hong SS, Kim YJ, Kim JK, Eun HW. Intraductal papillary mucinous neoplasm of the pancreas: Differentiate from chronic pancreatits by MR imaging. European Journal of Radiology. 2012;**81**:671-676

[52] Parakh A, Tirkes T. Advanced imaging techniques for chronic pancreatitis. Abdominal Radiology. 2020;**45**:1420-1438

[53] Graziani R, Frulloni L, Cicero C, Manfredi R, Ambrosetti MC, Mautone S, et al. Bull's-eye pattern of pancreatic-duct stones on multidetector computed tomography and gene-mutation-associated pancreatitis (GMAP). Radiological Medicine. 2012;**117**:1275-1286

[54] Luetmer PH, Stephens DH, Ward EM. Chronic pancreatitis: Reassessment with current CT. Radiology. 1989;**171**:353-357

[55] Yoon SH, Lee JM, Cho JY, Lee KB, Kim JE, Moon SK, et al. Small (≤ 20 mm) pancreatic adenocarcinomas: Analysis of enhancement patterns and secondary signs with multiphasic multidetector CT. Radiology. 2011;**259**:442-452

[56] Elbanna KY, Jang H-J, Kim TK. Imaging diagnosis and staging of pancreatic ductal adenocarcinoma: A comprehensive review. Insights into Imaging. 2020;**11**:58

Section 3

Anesthesiologist Perspective

Chapter 3

The Anesthesiologist Contribution to Management of Acute Pancreatitis

Annapaola Dotto

Abstract

Acute pancreatitis is a complex disease, and although most patients have a self-limiting illness, a minority of them develop severe disease and may need Intensive Care Unit admission. Regardless of severity degree, two cornerstones of acute pancreatitis multidisciplinary management are: fluid resuscitation and pain relief. These patients are frequently hypovolemic because of decreased oral intake, vomiting, fever, and fluid sequestration associated with pancreatic and systemic inflammation. Early intravenous volume resuscitation seems to reduce pancreatic hypoperfusion and multiorgan failure, but fluid overload has been associated with worse outcome, and maintaining proper hydration could be challenging. Acute pancreatitis is a very painful condition and effective analgesia is one of the priorities. Pain relief has a positive impact because of reduced stress response, sympathetic-induced vasoconstriction, and pulmonary complications. It is suggested to use a multimodal analgesic approach, to achieve patient's satisfaction, minimize opioid consumption and side effects. A modern and effective approach involves the use of patient-controlled analgesia and thoracic epidural analgesia. We would revise these two items to offer early and better multidisciplinary management to patients with acute pancreatitis, including those with mild to moderate disease, who are managed in general surgical wards, with the aim to improve their outcome and hospital stay.

Keywords: fluid resuscitation, systemic inflammatory response syndrome, pain management, epidural analgesia, patient-controlled analgesia

1. Introduction

Acute pancreatitis (AP) is an acute inflammatory disorder of the pancreas with a complex and variable course. Most patients develop only mild to moderate disease meaning no or just transient organ failure during the first 48 hours after the onset, but about 20–30% develops a severe form with local complications such as necrosis and often associated with single or multiple organs dysfunction and necessity of intensive care unit (ICU) admission. Severe AP is associated with persistent hemodynamic instability, respiratory distress with mechanical ventilation requirement, kidney failure, and is burdened by high mortality. ICU patients are often sedated and receive careful pain management, as well as careful hydration control [1, 2].

Patients with AP typically present with acute abdominal pain and significant depletion of intravascular volume. The main goal of initial treatment is to alleviate symptoms and prevent complications [3]. Fluid management and pain control are two central aspects of multidisciplinary care of AP, seem to impact on evolution, and influence the outcome. Management in the early hours gives the impression to be very important, when patients are usually assessed and assisted in the emergency department or general surgical ward.

Most patients have a self-limiting disease that resolves with supportive measures, and clinical choices can adjust the course of disease, reduce the hospitalization and health costs [4, 5].

Early intravenous volume resuscitation reduces pancreatic hypoperfusion and multiorgan failure, but fluid overload has been associated with worse outcome, and maintaining proper hydration could be challenging.

Pain relief has a positive impact because of reduced stress response, sympathetic-induced vasoconstriction, and pulmonary complications. A modern and effective multimodal analgesic approach aims to achieve patient's satisfaction and minimize side effects.

AP can evolve and worsen so it is required to routinely reassess the clinical parameters and personalize the fluidic and analgesic therapy [6].

There is evidence that the incidence of AP has been rising in recent years, probably due to the increase in the average age, obesity, and some drug therapy for chronic disease treatment too. As a result, they are patients with significant comorbidities that require a considerable health effort, which may involve several healthcare professionals.

This is why multidisciplinary management could be helpful, with the purpose of improving patient's outcome and hospital stay.

2. Fluid management

The AP treatment is currently symptomatic, and fluid management is a cornerstone of its therapy as well as being the intervention most likely to improve clinical outcomes. Patients are frequently hypovolemic due to decrease oral intake, vomiting, fever, tachypnea, and fluid sequestration associated with pancreatic and systemic inflammation. Pancreatic hypoperfusion may be attenuated by fluid resuscitation, therefore preventing pancreatic necrosis and lowering mortality [4, 7, 8].

Using experimental animal studies, it has been estimated that approximately two liters of fluid diffuse from the intravascular space to the interstitium, during the first 6 hours [7].

Fluid therapy to prevent hypovolemia and organ hypoperfusion comes from sepsis care, which has some pathophysiological similarities with AP.

After initial pancreatic acinar injury, the high amount of proteolytic enzymes produces local inflammation, proinflammatory cytokine, and vasoactive mediators release, with an increase in vascular permeability. Locally it results in interstitial fluid extravasation with edema of the gland, capillary vasoconstriction, and the production of microthrombi, which further worsen pancreatic perfusion. Cytokines such as interleukin (IL)-1, IL-6, IL-8 and systemic mediators such as tumor necrosis factor alpha (TNF-α) usually amplify this vicious circle and induce systemic inflammation, which can lead to systemic inflammatory response syndrome (SIRS).

SIRS is an exaggerated defense response of the body to a noxious stressor, which can be represented by infection, trauma, surgery, acute inflammation, ischemia, or reperfusion. Even though the purpose is defensive, the dysregulated cytokine storm can cause a massive inflammatory cascade leading to reversible or irreversible end-organ dysfunction and even death [9]. This storm represents the link between sepsis and AP, which is initially an aseptic inflammatory disease.

Likewise, as in septic patients, a low intravascular volume results in a decreased tissue perfusion, which can cause multiorgan failure, which increases complications and mortality rate. At the same time, overly aggressive hydration, especially in patients with preexisting kidney disease or hearth failure, increases the need for mechanical ventilation, the rates of infections, and thus mortality [1, 3].

Fluid dynamics are fundamentally different in mild and severe pancreatitis. The first one is easier to manage, because it is enough to restore the fluid deficit owing to vomiting, lower intake, and insensible losses. But the second one is characterized by vascular leakage with extravasation of protein-rich fluid, liquid sequestration, and hypoperfusion [10].

At the same time, we know that a mild form can evolve into a severe one, because in a sense they represent a pathophysiological continuum. Therefore, the revaluation is crucial to direct the right hydration and the evolution of the disease itself.

2.1 The fluid: How much of which one?

Unfortunately, there is still some degree of uncertainty about total amount of fluid, optimal infusion rate, and the type of solution.

Clinical data on the amount of fluid needed to prevent necrosis or to improve outcome are contradictory. In the past, an aggressive fluidic resuscitation meant a considerable and very rapid volume load, which could correspond of 2 liters bolus in the first hour and a subsequent maintenance of 20 ml/kg/h.

Even in some recent reviews, the initial volume of fluid administered varied substantially and also the strategy of maintenance—with or without initial bolus—was not uniform, with infusion's rates that vary from 1 to 15 ml/kg/h. Currently, however, it has emerged that a very early volume load in the course of AP may be beneficial, while rapid volume loads in advanced stages are harmful [7]. Hence, after fluid resuscitation in the first 12–24 hours, infusion should generally be curtailed, to avoid respiratory complications or abdominal compartment syndrome.

In fact, after 20–40 minutes of infusion, only 20% of crystalloid remains in the intravascular space because most inevitably migrates to the interstitium, further worsening the oxygen diffusion. This is why too much fluid is as harmful as too little.

The value of early goal-directed therapy in these patients remains unknown. It is evident that an excessively rigid protocol of fluid management is illogical because "one size doesn't fit all," while it may be more beneficial to identify some personalized therapeutic end points [4].

Intravascular volume and an adequate perfusing pressure need to be restored, but infusion rate should be carefully tailored to individual patients, considering factors such as age and comorbidities. Fluid resuscitation should focus on improving heart rate, mean arterial pressure, central venous pressure, urine output, blood urea nitrogen concentration, and serum lactate.

It appeared that colloid administration could improve the outcome. But actually hydroxyethyl starch (HES) fluids are not recommended in AP because subsequent studies failed to demonstrate improved mortality and instead found increasing rate of kidney injury or need for renal replacement therapy [11]. In fact, the American Gastroenterological Association (AGA) suggests against the use of HES fluids, however, with very low quality of evidence.

The use of high volumes of normal saline—0.9% sodium chloride—has also been shown to have harmful effects on plasma electrolyte balance, leading to hyperchloremic acidosis. The large chloride load results in acidosis that could promote or exacerbate inflammation and renal injury.

Now isotonic balanced crystalloids are the preferred fluid. Particularly strong evidences came from the SMART trial of 2018, which found a reduction rate of the composite outcome of death from any cause, new renal-replacement therapy, or persistent renal dysfunction in patients given balanced crystalloid than saline [6, 12].

A recent study indeed reports a shorter hospital stay and fewer ICU admissions in the group of patients randomized to receive Ringer's lactate, which is a balanced crystalloid isotonic versus plasma and seems to have an anti-inflammatory effect.

It is worth remembering that all these fluids are artificial solutions, which differ from human plasma composition. This is true also for balanced crystalloid, which varies in its electrolyte concentration, osmolality, and pH. Clinicians must then choose the better fluid to prescribe and its adequate amount, depending on the specific patient [13].

Based on multiple studies, a continuous infusion of 3 ml/kg/h would constitute aggressive and 1.5 ml/kg/h nonaggressive fluid therapy. As a general guidance, the choice of fluid should be a balanced crystalloid and the volume infused around 3–4 liters in the first 24 hours. There also should be predefined checkpoint at 6 or 8 hours to assess volemia and the other perfusion parameters [10, 14].

2.2 A rational strategy

As outlined before, initial management of AP within the first 48–72 hours of admission can modify the course of disease and length of hospital stay [5].

In the early phase, the goal is to restore circulating blood volume and improve peripheral tissue oxygenation. Easy clinical markers of adequate hemodynamic function are heart rate, blood pressure, respiratory rate, O_2 saturation, and urine output [8].

Fluid resuscitation is indicated to rapidly optimize tissue perfusion targets. In **Figure 1**, a practical approach is schematized, starting from resuscitation with 500–1000 ml of balanced crystalloid that is meant to normalize macrocirculation parameters such as blood pressure and heart rate and also microcirculation features such as refill time and skin color.

Obviously, this fluidic load is commensurate to the magnitude of hypotension and volume must be adjusted to the patient's age, weight, and preexisting renal injury or heart disease.

Subsequently, it is suggested to replace the ongoing losses with a continuous infusion of about 3 ml/kg/h during the first 12 hours and can be reduced to 1.5 ml/kg/h if physiological parameters improve or when patients resume hydration by mouth.

Caution is recommended to avoid fluid overload, and fluid administration should be guided by frequent reassessment of the hemodynamic status. However, it is particularly important to check blood pressure, heart rate, and pulse saturation every 6 or 8 hours, according to the severity of patient's disease, with the purpose of knowing if intravascular volume is adequate to ensure a good organ perfusion and oxygenation.

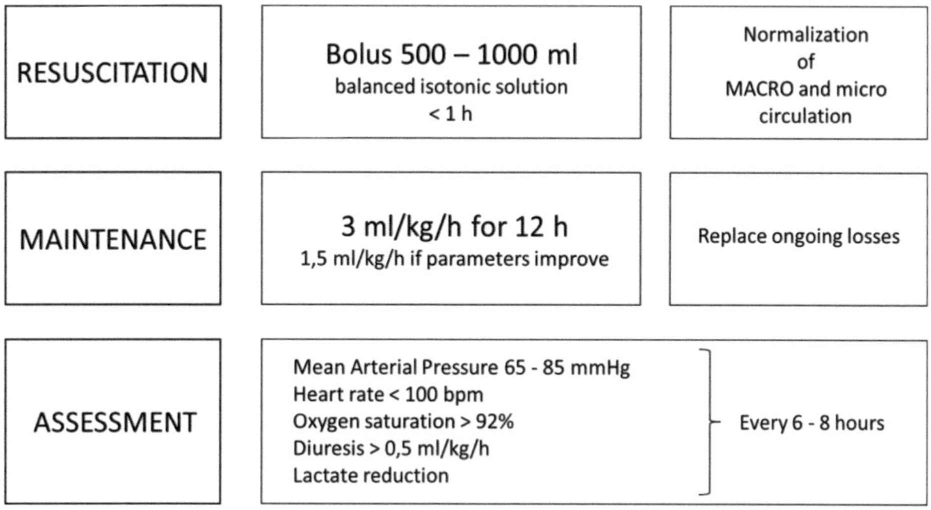

Figure 1.
Early fluid resuscitation strategy.

Most authorities recommend titrating intravenous fluids administration to specific measurable targets of perfusion, which in a nonintensive environment, may be well represented by effective diuresis and lactate reduction. These are two indicators of adequate organ perfusion and indirectly suggest that the availability of oxygen is appropriate [6].

It is extremely important to follow the evolution of the patient's clinical conditions to tailor our therapies. If there is no parameter improvement but rather diuresis contracts, lactates increase, respiratory insufficiency arises, or patient becomes hemodynamically unstable despite ongoing hydration, ICU transfer is indicated.

3. Pain control

Acute abdominal pain is the commonest presenting symptom of AP and the leading reason for hospital admission. It was already identified as the most popular finding by the board of International Symposium on Acute Pancreatitis of 1992 and still represents one of the three diagnostic criteria of the revised Atlanta Classification [15].

Pain consistent with AP is localized in the epigastric region and radiates like a belt around the trunk into the back. It is usually constant and described as deep and penetrating, due probably to retroperitoneal localization of pancreas. Pain may be exacerbated by eating, drinking, or lying supine and is often associated with nausea and vomiting [16, 17].

Its pathogenesis is complex and multifactorial: pancreatic acinar cell injury triggers the synthesis and release of pro-inflammatory cytokines and chemokines such as leukotrienes, bradykinin and arachidonic acid metabolites, and pancreatic proteases such as trypsin stimulate sensory neurons, which release substance P and calcitonin-gene-related peptide. This sophisticated signal net tends to self-amplify and involve the immune system with leukocytes activation too [18].

Whereas for almost all patients with AP experience pain, its relief is a clinical priority. Patients must receive satisfactory analgesia after hospital admission and until they need, tailored on subjective perception and modulated according with day-by-day pain variation, in order not to compromise their quality of life. Providing good analgesia is associated with enhanced lung function and reduced deep vein thrombosis: if pain is well controlled, patients can breathe deeply, sitting on chair and walking around. All these activities reduce length of stay and improve outcome.

Unfortunately, no guidelines provide sufficient details regarding analgesia administration in AP, and best current recommendation is to adhere to the acute pain management in the perioperative setting.

Several randomized controlled trials (RCTs) analyze the feasibility of a specific strategy or compare safety and efficacy of different analgesics, but clinicians who daily work in surgery or emergency wards probably do not find it very useful [19].

This is the reason why we revise the most recent literature and provide some simple indications about type, dose, route, and frequency of analgesia administration, in accordance with the current evidence.

3.1 Multimodal analgesia

Numerous studies have focused on comparing the efficacy of different classes of intravenous analgesic, in order to choose only one of these to manage AP pain, but a more modern approach is growing.

There is consistent evidence that multimodal analgesic approach should be used when treating postoperative pain, and it is possible to extend this concept to the management of acute pain in general, because it means achieve better pain control minimizing side effects. Combined different classes of analgesics such as nonsteroidal anti-inflammatory drugs (NSAIDs), paracetamol, and opioids, which act through several mechanisms and bind different receptors, enable to reach a satisfying analgesic plain, using a lower dose of each one [20].

NSAIDs inhibit prostaglandins production acting on phospholipase A2 and cyclooxygenases (COXs) and thus relieve pain by reduction of pro-inflammatory cytokines cascade. NSAIDs have been shown a protective effect against AP in elective contest such as endoscopic retrograde cholangiopancreatography (ERCP), probably because COX-1 and COX-2 inhibition downregulates local inflammation and mediators spread [21, 22].

Paracetamol is the most popular analgesic and antipyretic drug in the world and has the well-known advantage of being used even in patients at increased risk of bleeding, but its mechanism of action is still unclear. It has a central effect, when given as a rapid intravenous bolus over 15 minutes, which is mediated by serotoninergic descending pathway, inhibits cyclooxygenases (especially COX-3 isoenzyme), and acts via the endocannabinoid system. Therefore, its analgesic effect comes from a quite different process respect of NSAIDs and justifies their association [23].

Opioids are the most frequently prescribed analgesics for pain relief of patients with AP. All opioids used in clinical practice today exert their action on μ receptors, with some having additional activity on κ and δ. Opioid receptors are distributed throughout the central nervous system (CNS) and in the dorsal horn. They have two main effects: block incoming nociceptive afferents (medulla and brainstem) and increase the inhibitory activity of the descending pathways (periaqueductal gray). They act on multiple sites of the CNS, also lowering negative affective connotation of pain [24].

They are the most powerful analgesics available and beyond relieving pain they have the advantageous property of making patients feel relaxed and promote sleep.

People who are sick in fact are often distressed, anxious, insomnious because of discomfort, and sometimes oppositive to treatment.

Despite old beliefs about the risk of the Oddi's sphincter spasms after systemic administration, several studies have clarified that opioids do not negatively impact on the course of AP and could be safely administered, and their use may decrease the need for supplementary analgesia [25, 26].

It is known that opioids expose to a greater risk of nausea, vomiting, and stypsis and that is why the association with non-opioids helps to reduce the total amount of their administration but allowing to obtain an analgesia level that would be unthinkable with paracetamol alone.

No evidence or recommendation about any restriction in pain medication is available. Of course, NSAIDs should be avoided in patients with acute or chronic kidney injury.

Ensuring proper analgesia avoids the chronicization of pain and therefore the long-lasting intake of anti-inflammatory drugs or even worse opioids addiction.

Furthermore, pain is a potentially treatable cause of delirium, a condition that frequently affects elderly or multipathological patients admitted to hospital especially in the case of prolonged hospitalizations, as the case for AP in general. Delirium is an acute and fluctuating disturbance of consciousness with reduced ability to focus, maintain, or shift attention, accompanied by change in cognition. It includes psychomotor disturbances, disorder of the sleep–wake cycle, and emotional instability. It also causes poor patient cooperation, complicating medical and nursing care.

It is of clinical interest because it correlates with length of hospitalization, long-term cognitive dysfunction, and mortality; therefore, it is a costly health condition and significantly impacts on outcome and patient performance.

Delirium has multifactorial causes, but there is convincing evidence that sleep deprivation is a risk factor for the development and in our patients, insomnia is frequently pain-related [27].

3.1.1 A practical approach

Good pain management is providing timely coverage during all day. Both surgical and oncologic pain are controlled by prescription of one medication, or a combination of medications, that is given at regularly intervals through the day, for maximum control of baseline pain. This is the around-the-clock medication (ATC), and we could agree that a patient with AP deserve to receive at least paracetamol 1 g every 6 hours and one NSAIDs, for example, ketorolac 30 mg or ketoprofen 100 mg, every 8 hours (**Figure 2**) [28, 29].

In addition, we should also include a rescue therapy, to cover breakthrough pain that is not adequately covered by ATC and morphine 3 mg could be a good option because it's easily managed in the surgery ward and nursing staff are confident with. It is possible to administer again the same dosage after 30 minutes, which is the time for morphine to achieve maximum effect and the recommended dose is 10–15 mg within 24 hours, depending on the patient's age and kidney function. In fact, morphine has a long half-life and produces some active metabolites, and its elimination is dependent on kidney excretion, so it can easily accumulate in subjects with impaired renal function and cause undesirable effects such as respiratory depression. Old people are more sensitive to pharmacodynamic effect of opioids, and clinicians must be aware of this and pay more attention with their prescription [30].

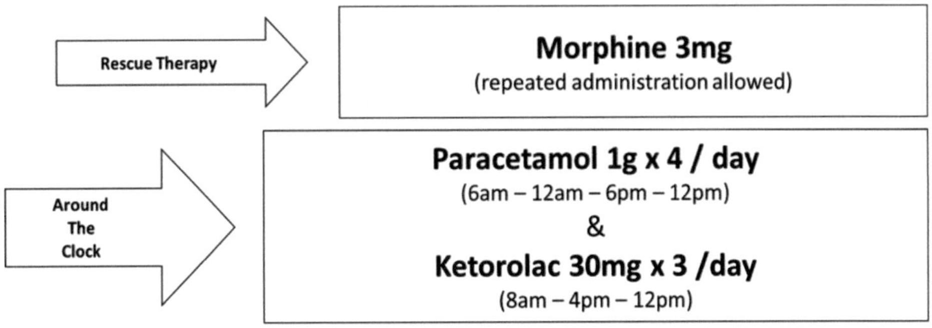

Figure 2.
An example of multimodal analgesia schematic approach.

Knowing that AP is an overly complex pathology and associated pain can range from mild to severe, it would be advisable to contact the anesthesiologist if the administered morphine exceeds 10 mg, because it might be reasonable to upgrade the analgesia strategy. A multidisciplinary approach to patient care is the key for a more comprehensive assessment and his greater satisfaction.

3.2 Patient-controlled analgesia

A patient-controlled analgesia (PCA) pump is a computerized machine that gives a programmed amount of analgesic, usually an opioid, when the patient presses a button (bolus or demand dose). The drug might be delivered only as a bolus, or also with a continuous background infusion (basal rate) depending on the pharmacokinetic and dynamic of the drug itself, the entity of pain, and the patient performance.

Anesthesiologist presets the dosage in order to make the infusion absolutely safe [31].

PCA is a widespread technique already used to treat acute and chronic pain, in postoperative setting and emergency department. It has proven to be more effective than non-patient opioid injections because patients can self-administer small dose of analgesic, this results in better pain control and higher satisfaction, moreover with a net reduction in opioid consumption [32].

It is universally recognized that undertreatment of pain has important impact, including hemodynamic fluctuation with tachycardia and hypertension, peripheral vasoconstriction, which can cause poor peripheral perfusion, activation of the stress response with increased cortisol production and hyperglycemia, and not least patient discomfort.

One of the problems with pain management is time from patient complain and drug administration. Unfortunately, sometimes it takes a lot because of department organization, and there is strong evidence that poorly controlled pain is much harder to relieve than and indeed increases the incidence of chronic pain.

PCA therapy increases patient satisfaction, decreases pain scores, and reduces opioid consumption [33, 34].

3.2.1 PCA with morphine

Morphine is used for the management of moderate to severe pain. It is metabolized in the liver with formation of several metabolites, among which morphine-6-glucuronide is actually responsible for the observed response. It is predominantly excreted

MORPHINE PCA				
Loading dose	**Bolus**	**Lockout**	**Continuous infusion**	**4-hour limit**
3–5 mg	1–3 mg	20 min	0.2– 0.5 mg/h	10–15 mg

Table 1.
Schematic morphine PCA administration.

in the urine, and its half-life elimination is about 2–4 hours, partly still under active metabolites. It is a drug with a high interindividual variability both as regards the pain reduction and side effects such as respiratory depression, constipation, nausea, and itching. Also for this it is important to choose an adequate administration protocol (**Table 1**) [35].

The bolus is the dose of morphine delivered each time the patient presses the button, and it might range from 1 to 3 mg depending on patient's physical characteristics: we will prefer lower dosages in elderly and frailty subjects. Morphine has an onset time of 15 minutes, but a slower peak effect, and it needs at least 30 minutes to exert its action. This is why the lockout interval, or time after a bolus in which another one is not allowed even if patient presses the button, is 20 minutes to permit the analgesic effect and prevent overdosing. Because of its long context-sensitive half time, after an adequate loading dose, the demand dose alone might be enough without background infusion, to reach satisfactory analgesia.

The 4-hour limit defines the maximum allowed amount of medication to be administered within that period, is usually less than the dose given if the patient presses the button every time, and acts as a safety mechanism.

The loading dose is a starting bolus that you can administer with the pump or manually with the aim to achieve more rapidly the patient well-being and having adequate stable concentration.

3.2.2 PCA with sufentanil

Among opioids, sufentanil has the highest therapeutic index, hence the safest to use. It is enormously powerful; therefore, it ensures excellent analgesia, but at the same time, it benefits from a much lower incidence of respiratory depression.

Is a highly lipophilic opioid and has a small volume of distribution. It has a time to peak effect after bolus of approximately 6–8 minutes, thus the patient will be able to manage in a satisfactory and punctual way his own analgesia, profiting from a rapid achievement of the effect.

It does not produce active metabolites and its excretion is not conditioned by renal function, as is the case for morphine, so it has a higher safety profile in elderly or patients with renal failure.

Its high therapeutic index and predictable pharmacokinetics make it the ideal candidate for administration via PCA pump as schematized in **Table 2** [36].

Sufentanil has a faster half-life of elimination than morphine and a sensitive context half-life that is too short, this is the reason why it is advisable to couple with a background infusion of about 2–5 μg/h to reach a stable concentration and maintain the analgesic effect between boluses. The continuous infusion will administer 72–120 μg in 24 hours, which represents a reasonable and harmless amount.

In most cases it may be enough to set a low infusion (2 μg/hour) and instead prefer a more consistent bolus (5 μg).

SUFENTANIL PCA				
Loading dose	**Bolus**	**Lockout**	**Continuous infusion**	**4 hours limit**
5–10 μg	2–5 μg	15 min	2–5 μg/h	40 μg

Table 2.
Schematic of sufentanil PCA administration.

The lockout may be shorter than what we usually set for morphine, because the sufentanil reaches peak effect more quickly, therefore 10–15 minutes are enough to ensure the effect perception, avoiding excessive self-administering.

It is preferable to give a loading dose before starting PCA infusion to immediately relieve patient's condition and maybe observe the effectiveness of it [37].

3.2.3 Ketamine

Ketamine is an old hypnotic that is back in vogue because at low concentration acts as a fantastically painkiller and has safe profile because it does not impact on respiratory drive.

It inhibits N-methyl-D-aspartate receptor (NMDA-R) of glutamate, which is the main excitatory neurotransmitter: blocks nociceptive peripheral afferents into posterior dorsal horn, propagation through spinal cord, brainstem. and then higher centers projections.

Ketamina acts synergistically with opioids and hence has an opioid-sparing effect. Blocking the NMDA receptor prevents the calcium channel opening and its entry into the cell, which would lead to a lowering of the pain threshold and a lack of pain control with opioids.

Adding a little amount of ketamine, for example, 40–50 mg, to the PCA pump could be an excellent way to improve the patient's analgesic management, reducing side effects and above all avoiding the need to increase morphine or sufentanil dosages. It also appears that this drug has the pleasant effect of mood improving, which can represent an added value to our therapy.

This approach significantly enhances activity of both morphine and sufentanil, improves their efficacy, and reduces tolerance to opioids [38–40].

3.3 Thoracic epidural analgesia

AP causes severe pain, which sometimes is difficult to adequately control with intravenous analgesics, therefore epidural analgesia becomes a good treatment option. Epidural analgesia is an essential component of perioperative medicine because it guarantees an excellent pain control, reduces opioid consumption, and improves recovery especially after major surgery. It is currently used for labor pain management in the delivery room because it allows to modulate analgesia according to the various stages of labor, with great mothers' satisfaction. It is also employed in ICU after severe chest trauma.

There is recent evidence from both preclinical and clinical trials supporting beneficial effects of epidural analgesia in AP. These studies suggest that epidural analgesia increases arterial perfusion of pancreas and redistribution of blood flow to nonperfused pancreatic regions [41, 42].

AP resulting from an inappropriate activation of trypsinogen leads to local injury and inflammation with increased capillary permeability, edema, augmented leukocyte adhesion, free radical production, and enhanced coagulation activity. This inflammatory vicious circle releases proinflammatory cytokines (IL-1, IL-6, IL-8) and systemic mediators (TNF-α) that discharge into the circulatory stream triggering a systemic inflammatory state.

Pancreatic tissue has been shown to be extremely sensitive to hypoxemia and ischemia, conditions that can lead to tissue necrosis and which strictly depend on microcirculation. Inadequate microvascular perfusion and hypoxia may play a significant role in early disease progression.

Thoracic epidural analgesia (TEA) induces a selective segmental sympathetic block, which, in addition of pain removal, increases splanchnic perfusion and reduces ischemic damage. TEA was found to improve gut mucosal perfusion and liver injury in sepsis too. It reduces pro-inflammatory state and improve outcome [43–45].

Significant complications related to the use of TEA are epidural hematoma, infection, and nerve damage. In spite of most of the research being done on patients admitted to ICU and thus with critical conditions, epidural has proved to be a safe technique [46]. This suggests that it can be used safely even in subjects with mild to moderate AP who are admitted to emergency or surgical department, if needed, for example, in obese or pneumopatic patients for whom we prefer to avoid opioids.

One of the reasons that creates reticence in the use of TEA is the fear of its hypotensive effect but, as for obstetrical analgesia, is possible to use low local anesthetics' concentrations with none or minimal hemodynamic impact.

3.3.1 Practical tips

Pancreas sympathetic afferent innervations originate from both thoracic and lumbar spinal cord (T6–L2 metamers). The epidural catheter might be placed at the thoracic level (indicatively between T8 and T10) and analgesia can be driven with an elastomeric continuous infusion or with a patient-controlled epidural analgesia (PCEA) with only mandatory bolus or demand dose.

In any case, the use of low anesthetic concentrations is recommended, for example, ropivacaine 0.05%–0.075% administered with bolus of 5–7 ml, to minimize the block extension regarding the risk of hypotension. If it is not enough to meet patient satisfaction, is possible to increase this concentration to 0.1%–0.125%. The association of an opioid is always indicated, and sufentanil 0.2–0.5 μg/ml may be a desirable choice because of is lipophilicity.

Combination with an opioid results in better analgesia with smaller dose of anesthetic [43].

3.4 Pain evaluation

A successful strategy of pain management starts with measuring the patient's pain.

The numeric rating scale (NRS) consists of a numeric version of the visual analog scale and is one of the most commonly used to assess pain severity (**Figure 3**). It helps healthcare professionals in quantifying a very subjective condition such as pain, in order to modulate analgesic administration and understand if current therapy works. On the other hand, it encourages patients to become active participants in pain assessment and management, and this is reflected on a well perception of care during hospital staying [47].

Scores also help in sharing information between different health professionals, speak the same language, and easily reassess patient's response.

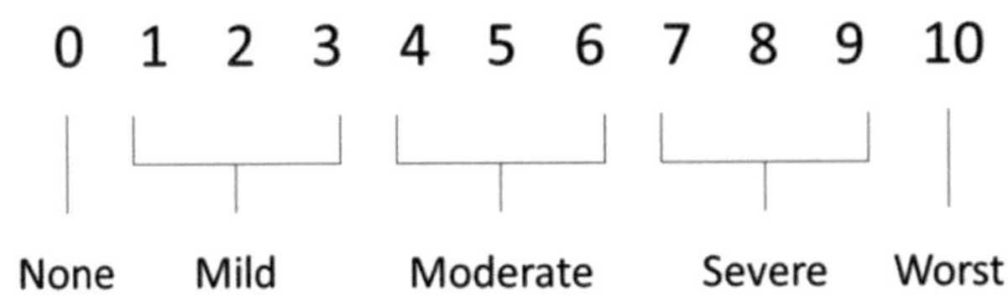

Figure 3.
Numeric rating scale.

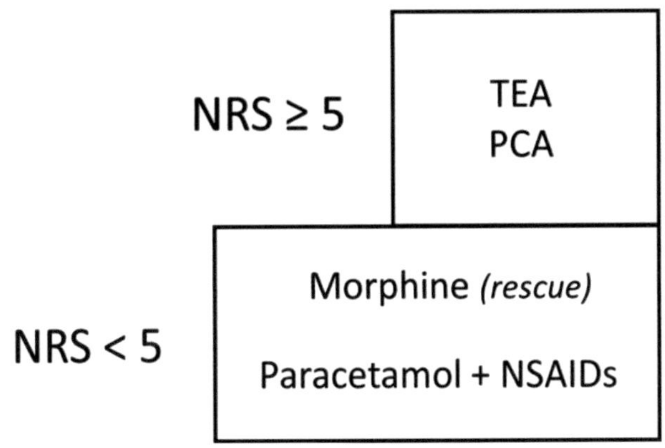

Figure 4.
Step up pain control.

NRS starts with zero that means no pain and well-being, numbers from 1 to 3 correspond to mild pain, from 4 to 6 moderate pain and above severe pain. Number 10 identifies worst possible pain.

3.4.1 The ladder and the clock

As mentioned above, not only is it important to ensure adequate analgesia during all phases of hospitalization, but also to choose the most appropriate strategy for the single patient.

The schematic approach in **Figure 4** suggests assessing NRS score of the patient and if it is inferior to 5, is possible to start with a simple intravenous analgesia round the clock at fixed hours. Instead, if NRS is more than 5, is better to choose a stronger approach like a pump or the epidural. So, it would be advisable to involve the anesthesiologist and planning the better strategy for the patient.

4. Conclusions

AP is a complex disease, and a growing understanding of its pathophysiology has proven that pancreatic microcirculation is crucial in the development of necrosis. Current evidence supports the benefit of a proper fluid administration and pain relief in optimizing tissue perfusion and reducing AP worsening.

Early fluid resuscitation is the key to optimize pancreatic perfusion, reduce local necrosis, prevent hemodynamic deterioration and the systemic impact of disease. At the same time, it is important not to overload the patient, because a fluid excess worsens the outcome.

Working as a multidisciplinary team allows to optimize patient management based on individual skill. With this in mind, anesthesiologists propose a more precise and modern approach to pain control with multimodal analgesia and step-up management with PCA and TEA.

A particularly important aspect of care is frequent reassessment of the patient's clinical conditions, physiological and humoral parameters, and even more considering their evolution trend, to tailoring fluid administration and analgesia.

Personalization of care not only improves outcome of patients, but also reduces their hospital stays.

Conflict of interest

None declared.

Thanks

Thanks to Dr. Antonio Farnia, for all his useful suggestions.

Author details

Annapaola Dotto
Department of Anesthesia and Intensive Care, Ca' Foncello Hospital – AULSS 2, Treviso, TV, Italy

*Address all correspondence to: annapaola.dotto@aulss2.veneto.it

References

[1] Mederos MA, Reber HA, Girgis MD. Acute pancreatitis: A review. JAMA. 2021;**325**(4):382-390. DOI: 10.1001/jama.2020.20317

[2] David Alter M et al. Comment & response: a review of acute pancreatitis to the editor. JAMA. 2021;**325**:2402-2404

[3] Goodchild G, Chouhan M, Johnson GJ. Practical guide to the management of acute pancreatitis. Frontline Gastroenterology. 2019;**10**(3):292-299. DOI: 10.1136/flgastro-2018-101102

[4] MacGoey P, Dickson EJ, Puxty K. Management of the patient with acute pancreatitis. BJA Education. 2019;**19**(8):240-245. DOI: 10.1016/j.bjae.2019.03.008

[5] Crockett SD et al. American Gastroenterological Association Institute guideline on initial management of acute pancreatitis. Gastroenterology. 2018;**154**(4):1096-1101. DOI: 10.1053/j.gastro.2018.01.032

[6] Leppäniemi A et al. 2019 WSES guidelines for the management of severe acute pancreatitis. World Journal of Emergency Surgery : WJES. 2019;**14**(1):1-20. DOI: 10.1186/s13017-019-0247-0

[7] Thomson A. Intravenous fluid therapy in acute pancreatitis: A critical review of the randomized trials. ANZ Journal of Surgery. 2018;**88**(7-8):690-696. DOI: 10.1111/ans.14320

[8] Stigliano S, Sternby H, de Madaria E, Capurso G, Petrov MS. Early management of acute pancreatitis: A review of the best evidence. Digestive and Liver Disease. 2017;**49**(6):585-594. DOI: 10.1016/j.dld.2017.01.168

[9] Chakraborty RK, Burns B. Systemic Inflammatory Response Syndrome. [Updated 2021 Jul 28]. In: StatPearls [Internet]. Treasure Island, Florida: StatPearls Publishing; Jan 2022

[10] Garg PK, Mahapatra SJ. Optimum fluid therapy in acute pancreatitis needs an alchemist. Gastroenterology. 2021;**160**(3):655-659. DOI: 10.1053/j.gastro.2020.12.017

[11] James TW, Crockett SD. Management of acute pancreatitis in the first 72 hours. Current Opinion in Gastroenterology. 2018;**34**(5):330-335. DOI: 10.1097/MOG.0000000000000456

[12] Semler MW et al. Balanced crystalloids versus saline in critically ill adults. The New England Journal of Medicine. 2018;**378**(9):829-839. DOI: 10.1056/nejmoa1711584

[13] Ostermann M, Randolph AG. Resuscitation fluid composition and acute kidney injury in critical illness. The New England Journal of Medicine. 2022;**386**(9):888-889. DOI: 10.1056/nejme2200294

[14] Lee A et al. Lactated ringers vs Normal saline resuscitation for mild acute pancreatitis: A randomized trial. Gastroenterology. 2021;**160**(3):955-957.e4. DOI: 10.1053/j.gastro.2020.10.044

[15] Bradley EL. Clinically based classification system for acute pancreatitis and regional complications. Problems in General Surgery. 1996;**13**(4):118-125

[16] Banks PA et al. Classification of acute pancreatitis - 2012: Revision of the Atlanta classification and definitions by international consensus. Gut.

2013;**62**(1):102-111. DOI: 10.1136/gutjnl-2012-302779

[17] De Jode LRJ. The management of acute pancreatitis. The British Journal of Clinical Practice. 1980;**34**(2):37-40. DOI: 10.3998/panc.2015.15

[18] Liddle RA, Nathan JD. Neurogenic inflammation and pancreatitis. Pancreatology. 2004;**4**(6):551-560. DOI: 10.1159/000082180

[19] Cai W et al. Pain Management in Acute Pancreatitis: A systematic review and Meta-analysis of randomised controlled trials. Frontiers in Medicine. 2021;**8**:1-13. DOI: 10.3389/fmed.2021.782151

[20] Helander EM, Menard BL, Harmon CM, et al. Multimodal Analgesia, Current Concepts, and Acute Pain Considerations. Current Pain and Headache Reports. 2017;**21**:3. DOI: 10.1007/s11916-017-0607-y

[21] Wu D, Bai X, Lee P, Yang Y, Windsor J, Qian J. A systematic review of NSAIDs treatment for acute pancreatitis in animal studies and clinical trials. Clinics and Research in Hepatology and Gastroenterology. 2020;**44**:100002. DOI: 10.1016/j.clirex.2019.100002

[22] Baxter KA et al. The effect of non-steroidal anti-inflammatory drugs on severity of acute pancreatitis and pancreatic necrosis. Annals of the Royal College of Surgeons of England. 2018;**100**(3):199-202. DOI: 10.1308/rcsann.2017.0205

[23] Przybyła GW, Szychowski KA. Paracetamol – An old drug with new mechanisms of action. CEPP Clinical and Experimental Pharmacology and Physiology. 2020;**2021**:3-19. DOI: 10.1111/1440-1681.13392

[24] Pathan H, Williams J. Basic opioid pharmacology: An update. British Journal of Pain. 2012;**6**(1):11-16. DOI: 10.1177/2049463712438493

[25] Basurto Ona X, Rigau Comas D, Urrútia G. Opioids for acute pancreatitis pain. Cochrane Database of Systematic Reviews. 2013;**7**:2013. DOI: 10.1002/14651858.CD009179.pub2

[26] Nelson AD et al. A systematic review and Meta-analysis of opioids vs nonopioids in acute pancreatitis. Gastro Hep Advances. 2022;**1**(1):83-92. DOI: 10.1016/j.gastha.2021.09.006

[27] Sampson EL, West E, Fischer T. Pain and delirium: Mechanisms, assessment, and management. European Geriatric Medicine. 2020;**11**(1):45-52. DOI: 10.1007/s41999-019-00281-2

[28] Inoue S, Miyoshi H, Hieda K, Hayashi T, Tsutsumi YM, Teishima J. Postoperative around-the-clock administration of intravenous acetaminophen for pain control following robot-assisted radical prostatectomy. Scientific Reports. 2021;**11**(1):1-7. DOI: 10.1038/s41598-021-84866-7

[29] Pasero C. Around-the-clock (ATC) dosing of analgesics. Journal of PeriAnesthesia Nursing. 2010;**25**(1):36-39. DOI: 10.1016/j.jopan.2009.12.003

[30] Glare PA, Walsh TD. Clinical pharmacokinetics of morphine. Therapeutic Drug Monitoring. 1991;**13**(1):1-23. DOI: 10.1097/00007691-199101000-00001

[31] Papa L, Maguire L, Bender M, Boyd M, Patel S, Samcam I. Patient controlled analgesia for the management of acute pain in the emergency department: A systematic review. The American Journal of Emergency Medicine. 2022;**51**:228-238. DOI: 10.1016/j.ajem.2021.10.042

[32] Mcnicol ED, Ferguson MC, Hudcova J. Patient controlled opioid analgesia versus non-patient controlled opioid analgesia for postoperative pain. Cochrane Database of Systematic Reviews. 2015;**6**:2015. DOI: 10.1002/14651858.CD003348.pub3

[33] Sinatra R. Causes and Consequences of Inadequate Management of Acute Pain. Pain Medicine. Dec 2010;**11**(12):1859-1871. DOI: 10.1111/j.1526-4637.2010.00983.x

[34] Downey LV, Zun LS. Pain management in the emergency department and its relationship to patient satisfaction. Journal of Emergencies, Trauma, and Shock. 2010;**3**(4):326-330. DOI: 10.4103/0974-2700.70749

[35] Hasslesstrom J, Sawe J. Morphine pharmacokinetics and metabolism in humans. Enterohepatic cycling and relative contribution of metabolites to active opioid concentrations. Clinical Pharmacokinetics. 2001;**40**(4):344-345

[36] Palmer PP, Miller RD. Current and developing methods of patient-controlled analgesia. Anesthesiology Clinics. 2010;**28**:587-599. DOI: 10.1016/j.anclin.2010.08.010

[37] Zhen L, Li X, Gao X, Wei H, Lei X. Dose determination of sufentanil for intravenous patient-controlled analgesia with background infusion in abdominal surgeries: A random study. PLOS ONE. 2018;**13**(10):e0205959. DOI: 10.1371/journal.pone.0205959

[38] Dahan A, Jonkman K, van de Donk T, Aarts L, Niesters M, van Velzen M. Ketamine for pain. F1000Research. 2017;**6**:1-8. DOI: 10.12688/f1000research.11372.1

[39] Balzer N, McLeod SL, Walsh C, Grewal K. Low-dose ketamine for acute Pain control in the emergency department: A systematic review and Meta-analysis. Academic Emergency Medicine. 2021;**28**(4):444-454. DOI: 10.1111/acem.14159

[40] Tseng W, Lin W, Lai H, Huang T, Chen P, Wu Z. A_randomized_controlled_study_.PDF. 2019;**28**

[41] Bulyez S et al. Epidural analgesia in critically ill patients with acute pancreatitis: The multicentre randomised controlled EPIPAN study protocol. BMJ Open. 2017;**7**(5):1-8. DOI: 10.1136/bmjopen-2016-015280

[42] Sadowski SM et al. Epidural anesthesia improves pancreatic perfusion and decreases the severity of acute pancreatitis. World Journal of Gastroenterology. 2015;**21**(43):12448-12456. DOI: 10.3748/wjg. v21.i43.12448

[43] Windisch O, Heidegger CP, Giraud R, Morel P, Bühler L. Thoracic epidural analgesia: A new approach for the treatment of acute pancreatitis? Critical Care. 2016;**20**(1):1-10. DOI: 10.1186/S13054-016-1292-7

[44] Harper D, McNaught CE. The role of thoracic epidural anesthesia in severe acute pancreatitis. Critical Care. 2014;**18**(1):1-2. DOI: 10.1186/cc13718

[45] Bachmann KA et al. Effects of thoracic epidural anesthesia on survival and microcirculation in severe acute pancreatitis: A randomized experimental trial. Critical Care. 2013;**17**(6):1-10. DOI: 10.1186/cc13142

[46] Jabaudon M et al. Thoracic epidural analgesia and mortality in acute pancreatitis: A Multicenter propensity analysis. Critical Care Medicine. 2018;**46**(3):e198-e205. DOI: 10.1097/CCM.0000000000002874

[47] Eriksson K, Wikström L, Årestedt K, Fridlund B, Broström A. Numeric rating scale: Patients' perceptions of its use in postoperative pain assessments. Applied Nursing Research. 2014;**27**(1):41-46. DOI: 10.1016/j.apnr.2013.10.006

Section 4

Endoscopic Features and Management

Chapter 4

Endoscopic Management of Acute and Chronic Pancreatitis

Stefano Benvenuti, Eleonora Pinese and Ilenia Barbuscio

Abstract

Acute pancreatitis (AP) is an inflammatory disorder of the pancreas, representing one of the most frequent causes of admission to hospital for gastrointestinal diseases in Western countries. Gallstones and alcohol play a fundamental role in the etiology of AP, but several other factors are involved, such as drugs, viruses, trauma, autoimmunity, anatomical anomalies. Chronic pancreatitis (CP) is a chronic inflammatory and fibrotic disease of the pancreas, in the pathogenesis of which both environmental factors, such as alcohol abuse and smoking, and genetic ones (SPINK1, CFTR, PRSS1 mutations) contribute. Endoscopic techniques are commonly used in the management of acute and chronic pancreatitis, allowing in many instances the avoidance of surgical intervention in acutely or chronically ill patients. This advantage is best represented by endoscopic removal of biliary stones in acute gallstone pancreatitis. Furthermore, also peripancreatic collections, such as pseudocyst or walled-off necrosis, can be managed endoscopically, ensuring a minimally invasive drainage. In CP endoscopy has a diagnostic role, especially in the early stages of the disease, but above all therapeutic, in the management of pancreatic duct strictures or stones. Other fields amenable to endoscopic intervention include treatment of potential causes of recurrent AP, such as sphincter of Oddi dysfunction and pancreas divisum.

Keywords: ERCP, EUS, walled-off necrosis, pseudocyst, acute pancreatitis, chronic pancreatitis

1. Introduction

Acute pancreatitis (AP) is an acute inflammatory process of the pancreas that may involve peripancreatic tissues and/or other remote organs, as part of a systemic inflammatory syndrome. It represents one of the most common causes of hospitalization for gastroenterological disorders [1].

The course of AP can be variable, with most patients showing a mild self-limited disease, requiring only supportive treatment. However, some patients still have a severe course, with a mortality rate of 10–20% [2]. Even if many factors, as intensive care unit intervention and early recognition and treatment of complications, have reduced mortality from AP over the past 20 years, the management of this disease remains challenging.

IntechOpen

Indication	Endoscopic therapy
Pain	
Pancreatic stone	ESWL, ERCP, per-oral pancreatoscopy (laser or electrohydraulic lithotripsy)
Pancreatic stricture	Stents (plastic or FCSEMS), EUS-guided drainage
Celiac plexus block	EUS-guided
Complication	
Biliary stricture	Stenting (multiple plastic stenting or FCSEMS)
Pseudocyst	Endoscopic drainage (EUS-guided, transpapillary, or combined)
Pancreatic duct leak	Transpapillary stenting
Vascular complications (gastric varices, pseudoaneurysm)	EUS-guided coil-glue, thrombin injection

ESWL, extracorporeal shock wave lithotripsy; ERCP, endoscopic retrograde cholangiopancreatography; FCSEMS, fully covered self-expandable metal stent; EUS, endoscopic ultrasonography.

Table 1.
Indications and endoscopic modalities in chronic pancreatitis.

The aims of endoscopy in AP include investigation and treatment of the causal factors and management of local complications, such as organized pancreatic necrosis, ductal disruption, and pseudocysts.

Chronic pancreatitis (CP) is a syndrome characterized by chronic progressive pancreatic inflammation, fibrosis, and scarring, resulting in damage and loss of exocrine (acinar), endocrine (islet cells), and ductal cells [3].

Pain is the predominant symptom observed during the course of CP. The etiopathogenesis of pain in CP is multifactorial and includes not only ductal hypertension due to obstruction of the pancreatic duct (PD) (calculi or stricture) but also neuropathy, peripheral sensibilization, and local or systemic complications (pseudocyst or distal biliary obstruction) [4]. Both pain intensity and frequency of pain attacks reduce quality of life in patients with CP.

Endoscopic therapy in painful CP is based on the rationale that pain is related to an overflow obstruction of the main pancreatic duct (strictures or pancreatic intraductal stones): the mainstay of endoscopic treatment includes decompression of pancreatic duct with stents (plastic or metal stent) in those with stricture(s), and fragmentation of pancreatic duct stone(s) using endoscopic retrograde cholangiopancreatography (ERCP) and/or in combination with extracorporeal shock wave lithotripsy (ESWL). This is the reason why only selected cases of patients with CP are amenable to endoscopic treatment.

Endoscopic ultrasonography (EUS) has emerged as a complementary endoscopic modality in the management of CP as well as associated complications like pseudocysts, refractory pain, and vascular complications (**Table 1**).

2. Acute pancreatitis

2.1 Endoscopic management of acute biliary pancreatitis

In Western countries, gallstone represents the first cause of AP, accounting for almost half of the cases, affecting middle-aged people, especially women [5].

The pathogenic mechanism by which gallstones determine AP is a temporary obstruction of the main pancreatic duct. Biliary AP should be suspected in presence of elevated liver function tests (LFTs) within 24–48 hours of the onset of symptoms, with alanine aminotransferase (ALT) >3× upper limit of normal having a 95% positive predictive value for AP. Nevertheless, its negative predictive value is only 50%. Aspartate aminotransferase (AST), alkaline phosphatase (ALP), and bilirubin have both low sensitivity and negative predictive value [6].

Most patients with biliary AP have a mild-to-moderate disease course, benefiting from conservative management. The majority of common bile duct (CBD) stones causing biliary AP are small (≤5 mm), and their spontaneous passage into the duodenum occur in 80% of cases, with no need for endoscopic intervention. Magnetic resonance imaging (MRI) or EUS is requested to exclude the presence of CBD stones, prior to ERCP. While the utility of EUS in identifying the cause of AP after the acute attack is well established, data regarding the role of EUS during hospitalization for AP are limited. In presence of AP edema of the duodenal wall, pancreatic and peripancreatic inflammation, fluid or necrotic collections make difficult the study of pancreatic parenchyma, gallbladder, and biliary tree. Thus, EUS aimed to identification of small pancreatic cancer or early changes of chronic pancreatitis must be avoided. On the contrary, EUS could be useful in the diagnosis of choledocholithiasis due to its higher sensitivity compared to MRCP for small CBD stones (<5 mm). In those patients with AP and intermediate risk of CBD stones, EUS may avoid unnecessary ERCP [7, 8].

Guidelines recommend against urgent ERCP (within 48 hours) in AP, especially in case of severe disease, unless in presence of cholangitis or ongoing/worsening biliary obstruction. However, if choledocholithiasis is confirmed, ERCP with biliary sphincterotomy and stones extraction should be performed during the index hospitalization, in order to reduce the rate of readmission for a new episode of biliary AP. If CBD has been completely cleared from stones during ERCP, biliary stenting is not routinely indicated before cholecystectomy. In cases of acute suppurative cholangitis, when smaller contrast injection and shorter procedural time, due to bad clinical status of the patient, are required, placement of a biliary stent can ensure adequate drainage, waiting to be able to perform biliary stone extraction. In patients with large bile duct stones, endoscopic large balloon dilation after sphincterotomy is suggested [9].

In case of mild biliary AP, same-admission cholecystectomy or early cholecystectomy (within 2–4 weeks from the onset of AP) is recommended, to avoid recurrence of AP [10].

2.2 Endoscopic management of acute pancreatitis associated with congenital variants

2.2.1 Pancreas divisum

Pancreas divisum (PD) represents the most frequent congenital pancreatic malformation, resulting from a failure of the fusion between dorsal and ventral pancreatic ducts during the second month of fetal life, with preferential pancreatic juice outflow via the dorsal pancreatic duct through the minor papilla. PD is defined as complete if no communication between the ventral and dorsal ducts is visible, incomplete if communication remains. The prevalence of PD in caucasian population is about 5–10%, and more than 95% of these patients are asymptomatic, with incidental diagnosis on abdominal imaging [11].

PD has long been regarded as a predisposing factor to AP, but studies conducted on individuals with recurrent AP showed that the comparable AP incidence between patients with PD and those with normal ductal anatomy. PD is, infact, a co-factor which in association with certain genetic mutations of serine protease inhibitor Kazal type 1 (SPINK1) gene, cystic fibrosis transmembrane conductance regulator (CFTR) gene, and chymotrypsin C (CTRC) gene increases the risk of AP [12]. Other additional factors that can determine AP in PD are the presence of stenosis of the minor papilla or santorinicele, which consists in cystic dilatation of the distal dorsal duct just proximal to the minor papilla [13].

ERCP is the gold standard for diagnosis of PD, but it is not used as a diagnostic method, given its invasiveness and the high accuracy of magnetic resonance pancreatography after secretin injection (s-MRCP) [14]. EUS shows also a high diagnostic accuracy for PD with a sensitivity of 87–95%, with absence of a "stack sign," i.e., the parallel alignment of distal CBD, ventral pancreatic duct and portal vein, presence of a "crossed duct sign," which is given by the crossing of dorsal pancreatic duct over the bile duct anteriorly and superiorly [15].

In asymptomatic patients with incidental diagnosis of PD therapeutic measures are not required, reserving them for those with recurrent attacks of AP, even if of mild entity, or those who had one attack of severe AP in absence of other identifiable causal factors. Also the presence of santorinicele with large main pancreatic duct could be an indication for treatment. Endoscopic therapy includes minor papilla endoscopic sphincterotomy (mPES) and minor papilla orifice balloon dilation. Given the high risk of post-ERCP AP associated with both these procedures, placement of a prophylactic temporary pancreatic stent is advisable [16].

2.2.2 Other congenital variants

Anomalous pancreatobiliary union (ABPU) affects 1.5–3% of individuals, and it consists in the union of the pancreatic and bile ducts outside the duodenal wall, resulting in a longer common channel (more than 15 mm proximal to the duodenum) that promotes reflux of bile and pancreatic juice into the alternative duct. Therefore, stones, protein plugs, or sphincter of Oddi dysfunction can cause temporary obstruction to pancreatic flow. All these factors determine an increase of pancreaticobiliary intraductal pressure, leading to AP [17]. AP is reported in 3–31% of APBU patients, and it is generally mild and self-limiting. Endoscopic sphincterotomy may decrease the risk of AP in these patients [18].

Choledochocele is a rare congenital or acquired condition, consisting in dilatation of the intraduodenal segment of the CBD. In these patients, AP occurs when the cystic dilatation or its content (sludge or stones) causes obstruction of the pancreatic duct outflow. Endoscopic sphincterotomy in order to unroof the choledochocele is recommended [19].

2.3 Endoscopic management of acute idiopathic pancreatitis

Recurrent AP is defined by the occurrence of two or more episodes of AP. Etiological diagnosis of AP is achieved in 70–90% of cases. Minimal diagnostic workup during a first episode of acute pancreatitis is suggested by guidelines and includes detailed personal history, family history, physical examination, laboratory tests (i.e. liver enzymes, calcium, and triglycerides), and transabdominal ultrasound (US) [20]. If etiology cannot be determined using this workup, AP is defined idiopathic, and this occurs in around 10–30% of cases [21].

There are several causes of AP that may be missed with this workup, and thus further diagnostic modalities, such as MRCP and computed tomography (CT), should be considered to rule out the presence of ductal adenocarcinoma or intraductal papillary mucinous tumors, or autoimmune pancreatitis. EUS may identify an etiology in 61% idiopathic AP, mainly represented by microlithiasis or sludge [22]. Also early chronic pancreatitis could be diagnosed with EUS, as possible cause of recurrent AP. When no etiologic factors are identified, sphincter of Oddi dysfunction should be suspected. ERCP with sphincter of Oddi manometry is the gold standard diagnostic test, but it is associated with significant morbidity [23]. At present, ERCP with sphincterotomy represents the treatment of choice for patients with structural or functional stenosis of the sphincter of Oddi, with reports of 70–90% resolution of symptoms [24].

2.4 Endoscopic management of acute pancreatitis complications

2.4.1 Pancreatic fluid collections

Pancreatic fluid collections (PFCs) are a frequent complication of AP, and their correct classification is important to guide the management. In 2012, an international working group has modified the Atlanta classification for AP, introducing new terminology for PCFs, which are classified according to the time elapsed since the collection was formed and to the presence or absence of necrosis. Acute collections in the first 4 weeks are called acute necrotic collections (ANCs) if necrosis is present or acute peripancreatic fluid collections (APCs), in absence of necrosis. After 4 weeks, when a capsule develops, persistent acute peripancreatic fluid collections are called pseudocysts and acute necrotic collections are called walled-off necrosis (WON) (**Figure 1**) [25]. The majority of APC resolve spontaneously and only a 5–15% of them transform into pseudocyst. On the contrary, half of ANC become WON. 16–47% of pancreatic necrosis get infected [26, 27].

PFCs drainage is recommended in presence of symptoms and/or complications such as abdominal pain, gastrointestinal obstruction, vascular compression, biliary obstruction, or infection. Size alone is not an indication for treatment. Historically, drainage has been performed via surgical techniques. However, in the last decade,

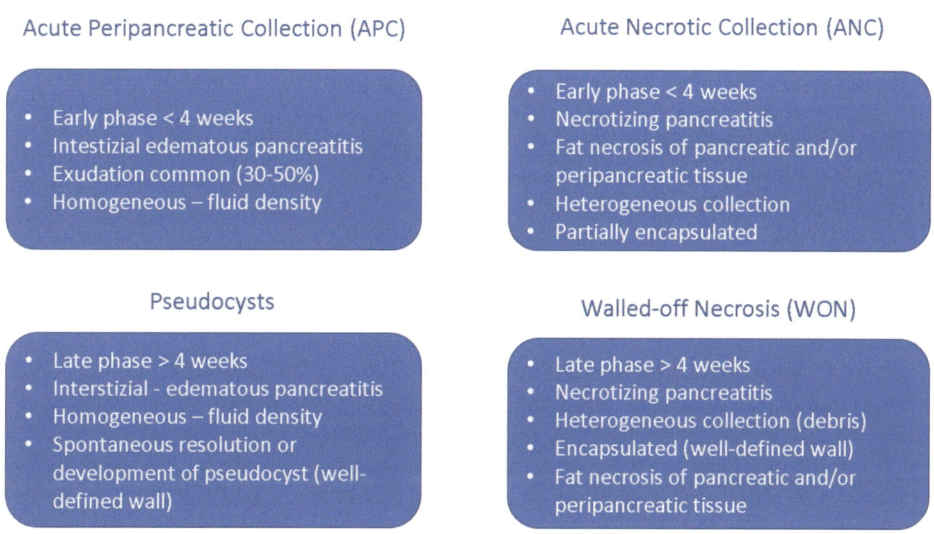

Figure 1.
Pancreatic fluid collections.

thanks to new and advanced endoscopic tools and expertise and consequent reduction in health care costs, minimally invasive endoscopic drainage has become the preferable approach [28].

The first conventional endoscopic transmural drainage of PFCs consisted of endoscopic visualization of PFC bulge in the gastric wall, creation of a fistulous tract between PCF and gastric lumen with a seldinger technique, insertion of a guidewire into the PFCs cavity, dilation of the tract, and, finally, deployment of one or more plastic stents to secure apposition of the lumens and continuous drainage [29]. A nasocystic catheter was generally performed to promote liquefaction of the debris and improve drainage. Infusion of hydrogen peroxide (H_2O_2) facilitated dislodgement and removal of necrotic debris. Adverse events, even if rare, such as bleeding, perforation, and self-limited pneumoperitoneum, have been reported [30]. To remedy the suboptimal drainage efficiency of plastic stents, especially in WON, covered biliary metal stents were used for this purpose. However, they were associated with complications, such as migration, erosions, or ulceration over gastric or retroperitoneal side and difficulty in performing necrosectomy [31].

Recently, a new dedicated bi-flanged lumen apposing metal stent (LAMS) has been introduced for EUS drainage of PFCs. LAMS has been specifically designed to create an anastomosis between the cyst cavity and the gut lumen. At first, the insertion of a guidewire inside the collection by a standard 19G FNA needle was necessary to release the stent. Subsequently, a new device in which the LAMS is equipped with an electrocautery-enhanced delivery system avoided the use of multiple accessories to achieve the drainage. Different diameters are available for these stents [32]. Published data report that, compared to plastic stents and fully covered metal biliary stents, LAMS determines an earlier resolution of PFCs. They are associated with increased costs and, in the first published series, with increased risk of adverse events, in particular pseudoaneurysm-related bleeding [33]. Recent studies have shown that earlier removal of LAMS, within 3 weeks from stent placement, significantly reduces the frequency of bleeding complications, with same rate of adverse events of plastic stents. Finally, recent scientific literature supports the use of LAMS for drainage of PFCs, mostly because they make possible to access the WOPN cavity with a standard gastroscope, after dilatation of the cysto-gastric tract with a balloon, to perform lavage and direct endoscopic necrosectomy (DEN) [34]. Hydrogen peroxide plus normal saline is used for the lavage of the cavity, and then necrotic debris is removed under direct vision using snares or baskets. Several sessions may be necessary to achieve complete DEN.

2.4.2 Disconnected pancreatic duct syndrome

In severe AP, necrosis of the pancreatic parenchyma may cause loss of integrity of the pancreatic duct, determining duct disruption, i.e., a partial interruption of the duct integrity, or its disconnection, i.e., a circumferential interruption of the duct. This leads to extraductal and extrapancreatic leakage, which can be complicated by recurrent PCFs and their possible infection, or pancreatic fistulas [35].

The diagnosis of disconnected pancreatic duct syndrome (DPDS) is usually delayed, given a lack of awareness on the topic, resulting in increased morbidity, cost of treatment, and duration of hospital stay. Surgery has been for long time the best approach for the management of DPDS, consisting of either resection or internal drainage procedures. Anyway, in the setting of a severe AP, surgery is often difficult due to presence of local inflammation and vascular alterations, as extensive venous collaterals consequent to splenic vein thrombosis [36]. With recent advancements, endoscopy offers new minimally invasive therapeutic options for the management of DPDS. When a co-existent PFC is present, endoscopic approach consists of EUS-guided transmural drainage. In DPDS without a co-existing PFC, surgery is the best option as endoscopy cannot ensure internal drainage of the secretions of disconnected pancreas. Transpapillary drainage in patients with is effective only in patients with partial pancreatic duct disruption that can be bridged with the positioning of a stent. In complete disruption of pancreatic duct, bridging with pancreatic stent is often not feasible [37].

3. Chronic pancreatitis

3.1 Endoscopic diagnosis of chronic pancreatitis

Diagnosis of CP derives from a combination of clinical symptoms, as abdominal pain, malabsorption, diabetes mellitus, and pancreatic function tests, as fecal elastase and morphological pancreatic abnormalities, and as calcifications, atrophy, ductal dilatation or strictures, and pseudocysts. At advanced stages of the disease, when both symptoms and morphological alterations are present, reaching the diagnosis is generally easy. On the contrary, it is much more challenging in earlier stages, given both to the low sensitivity and specificity of usual diagnostic methods and to the absence of a widely shared definition of early CP. According to a recent consensus, the term "early" describes the disease state rather than the disease duration; thus, it refers to a condition in which features of advanced CP are lacking [38].

Imaging has a fundamental role in the diagnosis and therapeutic management of patients with CP, and the most frequently used imaging modalities for CP are EUS, ERCP, MRI, computed tomography (CT), and abdominal ultrasound (US). EUS and ERCP showed the highest sensitivity (81 and 82%, respectively) and specificity (90 and 94%, respectively) [39]. Nevertheless, guidelines recommend using US, CT, and MRI as first imaging diagnostic approach, due to their larger availability and noninvasiveness, reserving EUS only to cases in which cross-sectional imaging is not conclusive [40]. ERCP should be used for therapeutic purposes only.

EUS diagnosis of CP is based on the assessment of ductal and parenchymal morphologic features, which correspond to histopathological changes. They initially embraced 11 criteria, then become 9, which are summarized in **Table 2**. In the absence of any criteria, a diagnosis of chronic pancreatitis is unlikely, whereas when five or more criteria out of nine are present, chronic pancreatitis is likely [41].

Since the different pathological characteristics in CP have not the same importance in terms of diagnostic value, the "nine criteria classification," giving to each criterion the same relevance, has not a high diagnostic accuracy. Thus, another scheme,

Parenchymal abnormalities	Ductal abnormalities
Hyperechoic foci with and without shadows	Stones in the duct
Hyperechoic strands	Duct irregularity
Cysts	Main duct dilation
Honeycomb-like lobulation	Visible side branches
	Hyperechoic contours on the main duct

Table 2.
Nine classic criteria for establishing a diagnosis of chronic pancreatitis on EUS.

Major A criteria: • Hyperechoic features with shadowing • Main pancreatic duct calcifications
Major B criteria: • Lobularity with honeycombing
Minor criteria • Lobularity without honeycombing • Hyperechoich features without shadowing • Pseudocysts • Stranding • Irregular main pancreatic duct • ≥ Dilated duct branches • Main pancreatic duct dilation • Hyperechoic main pancreatic duct wall

Table 3.
The Rosemont classification for endoscopic ultrasound-based criteria for the diagnosis of chronic pancreatitis.

named Rosemont classification, proposed by the International Consensus, divides parenchymal and ductal criteria in major and minor features. Major criteria for CP are hyperechoic foci with shadowing and main pancreatic duct (PD), calculi and lobularity with honeycombing. Minor criteria for CP are cysts, dilated ducts, irregular pancreatic duct contour, dilated side branches, hyperechoic duct wall, strands, non-shadowing hyperechoic foci, and lobularity with noncontiguous lobules (**Table 3**) [42]. Basing on these consensus criteria, the EUS diagnosis could be consistent with CP, suggestive of CP, indeterminate for CP or normal (**Table 4**).

3.2 Endoscopic management of obstructive pancreatic ductal stone

Pancreatic stones seem to arise either as direct and evenly calcified stones or as radiolucent protein plugs that may or may not become calcified during the course

Consistent with CP A. 1 major A feature (+) ≥ 3 minor features B. 1 major A feature (+) major B feature C. 2 major A features
Suggestive of CP A. 1 major A feature (+) <3 minor features B. 1 major B feature (+) ≥3 minor features C. ≥5 minor features (any)
Indeterminate for CP A. 3 to 4 minor features, no major features B. Major b features alone or with <3 minor features
Normal ≤ 2 minor features, no major features

Table 4.
EUS diagnosis of CP on the basis of consensus criteria.

of the disease [43]. The majority of pancreatic stones are calcified and radiopaque. Their prevalence increased with time and was detected in approximately 62% of patients with CP [44]. The best candidates for the successful treatment of painful CP are patients with solitary stones, with distal obstruction of the main pancreatic duct (located in the pancreatic head), and with a mean size of 10 mm and associated with strictures [4, 45].

ERCP and extraction are recommended for smaller (< 5 mm), nonimpacted stones of the main pancreatic duct [46]. ERCP can achieve main pancreatic duct drainage by sphincterotomy of the major and/or minor papilla, by short-term stent placement, or by pancreatic stone extraction using basket or balloon. Endoscopic therapy is also preferable in patients with risk factor (older age, co-morbidities) instead of surgery.

ESWL is recommended for fragmentation of large (> 5 mm), radiopaque stone(s) located preferentially in the pancreatic head [45]. For radiolucent calculi (difficult to target with X-ray), a nasopancreatic tube can be placed to facilitate targeting of the stones during ESWL [47].

Endoscopy alone allows stone extraction in a minority of CP patients (9–14%) [48, 49]; ESWL prior to endoscopy therapy allowed extraction of pancreatic stone in >80% of patients after failed stone extraction at primary endoscopy [48]. Pancreatic mechanical lithotripsy is burdened by major complications compared to biliary mechanical lithotripsy, and these included trapped or broken basket, traction wire fracture, and pancreatic ductal leak.

Pancreatic stone fragmentation after ESWL is obtained in 90% of patients (after multiple sessions) [50].

In a recent meta-analysis, ESWL alone allowed complete/partial main pancreatic duct clearance in 70%/22% of patients, respectively; pain was absent or mild–moderate during the 2 years following treatment in 52.7% and 33.4% of patients, respectively; quality of life improved in 88.2% of patients [51].

ESWL in not free from complications: most frequent is pancreatitis (up to 4.2%). The most severe complications are infection, acute stone incarceration in the papilla, bleeding, and perforation. Other minor adverse events reported are asymptomatic hyperamylasemia, hematuria, gastrointestinal mucosal injury, skin erythema, and tenderness in the region of contact with the shockwave head [52].

The systematically addition of endoscopic therapy after ESWL is not recommend by the European Society of Gastrointestinal Endoscopy (ESGE) [45]. Some studies and retrospective series reported similar decreases in main pancreatic duct diameter and no differences in pain resolution, instead of longer hospital stay and higher costs for patients who had ESWL combined with ERCP [53, 54].

Per-oral pancreatoscopy (POP)-assisted electrohydraulic lithotripsy (EHL) or laser lithotripsy (LL) is an emerging technology to fragment large intraductal stone(s). In a recent review and meta-analysis, technical success and overall fragmentation success were 91.2% and 85.5%, respectively [55]. Furthermore, stone fragmentation and ductal clearance could be achieved in 62% of patients in a single session; this suggests that POP may be an effective alternative to ESWL. Currently, with the newer version of cholangioscopes (SpyGlass-DS, Boston Scientific, Marlborough, MA), this technique will increase in the next few years.

The safety of POP-guided lithotripsy has been confirmed in two systematic reviews [55, 56]. The most common adverse events were post-ERCP pancreatitis (7%), pain (4.7%), perforation (4.3%), and hemorrhage (3.4%); overall, the incidence of adverse events was 11.2% with EHL and 13.1% with LL. Moreover, the technique has many advantages: it allows direct visualization of the stones (reducing ductal injury), it can identify radiolucent stones, and it can confirm ductal clearance after lithotripsy [57]. However, the weaknesses of POP include need of expertise, additional costs, and need to dilated pancreatic duct (to allow insertion of pancreatoscope).

ESGE suggests to consider POP-guided lithotripsy when ESWL is not available or for stones that were not fragmented after adequately performed ESWL [45].

3.3 Endoscopic management of pancreatic stricture

Strictures of the main pancreatic duct may be a complication of a previously embedded stone or a consequence of acute inflammatory changes around the main pancreatic duct [58]. Strictures may be classified as either nondominant or dominant. Dominant main pancreatic duct strictures are defined by the presence of at least one of the following characteristics: 1) upstream main pancreatic duct dilatation (≥6 mm in diameter), 2) prevention of contrast medium outflow beside a 6-Fr catheter inserted upstream from the stricture, and/or 3) abdominal pain during continuous infusion of a nasopancreatic catheter inserted upstream from the stricture with 1 L saline for 12–24 h [45, 59].

Before endoscopic treatment of man pancreatic duct strictures, malignancy should be excluded, by cross-sectional imaging and cytology brushing (especially for patients without pancreatic calcification) [60].

Endoscopic management of pancreatic duct stricture includes pancreatic sphincterotomy, dilatation of the stricture using bougie, balloon or Soehendra stent retriever, followed by placement of one or multiple plastic stents [61]. Technical success is defined by stent insertion across a dominant main pancreatic duct stricture (or most proximal one in case of multiple strictures), and it aims to 1) decompress the main pancreatic duct and improve pain and 2) dilate the stricture(s). Less frequent indication includes facilitation of main pancreatic duct stone clearance in association with ESWL [62].

Dominant strictures are single in >80% of the patients, and insertion of single 10-Fr plastic stent can be used as the initial endoscopic therapy. In responders, endotherapy should be continued for at least 1 year before permanently removing the stent. Stent should be replaced if necessary (every 6 month or on demand), based on symptoms or signs of stent dysfunction [45].

Stricture resolution was achieved in 9–50% of patients [58, 63]; long-term pain relief is experienced by about two-thirds of patients (67.5%) after stenting. However, resolution of the stricture after stent removal was observed only in a minority of patients [64]. The follow-up after stent removal in most study was >24 months.

Refractory pancreatic duct stricture is defined as a symptomatic dominant stricture that persists or relapses after a single pancreatic stent placement indwelling for 1 year [45]. A substantial proportion of pancreatic duct stricture may not respond to conventional endoscopic therapy (single plastic stent). Treatment options for these strictures are multiple side-by-side plastic stents, self-expandable metal stents (SEMSs), or surgery. The use of multiple plastic stenting during multiple sessions of endotherapy allowed stricture resolution in 89.5% of patients and pain relief in 77.1% of patients after 9.5 years follow-up [65, 66].

More recently, the use of SEMS and biodegradable stents has been described for refractory pancreatic strictures. With respect to SEMS, only fully covered SEMS (FCSEMS) has provided acceptable results: pain improvement in 37–88% of patients (follow-up of 3–4 years) [67, 68]. However, there were no differences in pain relief between multiple plastic stenting and FCSEMS (84.2% vs. 85.2%). The main advantage of FCSEMS over multiple stenting is a lower number of endoscopic sessions [69].

Regarding complication with plastic stent, the most commonly reported in the short term were mild pancreatitis (severe pancreatitis was very rare) or worsening of pancreatic pain, followed by sepsis (2.6%), cholangitis (2.3%), and post-sphincterotomy bleeding (1.5%). During follow-up, distal (3.6%) or proximal (2.7%) stent migration and stent obstruction (almost all stent become obstructed for3 months) are reported. Furthermore, stent-induced ductal lesions were described in 18% of patients and mortality in 0.4% [45].

Adverse events reported with the use of FCSEMS include pain (7–20%), stent migration (15–46%), de novo strictures (16–27%), pancreatitis, cholestasis, and cholangitis [45, 70].

In symptomatic patients with main pancreatic duct obstruction and failure of conventional transpapillary drainage, endosonography-guided (EUS-guided) therapy can be a chance. The technic consists of puncturing the main pancreatic duct through duodenal or gastric wall, and a guidewire is inserted in the pancreatic duct to proceed with transpapillary (rendezvous technique) or transmural drainage using a stent [71]. This is a difficult technique that should be performed only in tertiary centers after multidisciplinary discussion [45]. In successful procedure, immediate pain relief has been reported in a majority of patients (50–100%); during long-term follow-up, pain relief was achieved in 70–90% of patients. In large series, failure of EUS-guided technique occurs approximately in 10% of cases and complications occur in about 10% that include severe pancreatitis, bleeding, hematoma, and perforation [72, 73]. Frequently (20–55%), stent migration or occlusion needs endoscopic reintervention.

3.4 Endoscopic management of chronic pancreatitis complications

3.4.1 Biliary stricture

Biliary strictures occur in about 10–15% of patients with CP [74]. Strictures can be asymptomatic or present with jaundice, cholangitis, choledocholithiasis, or asymptomatic elevation of ALP and/or bilirubin [75]. Before endoscopic treatment, malignancy should be reasonably excluded.

Biliary strictures related with CP are resistant to endoscopic treatment due to periductal fibrosis and calcification [74]. Endoscopic treatment consists of an ERCP with stent(s) placement to achieve biliary decompression. Only a small percentage of patients respond to a single plastic stent placement [76]. The suggested approach for benign biliary stricture consists of temporarily dilating the stricture using multiple side-by-side plastic stents (exchange every 3–6 months) or FCSEMS [77, 78]. Both approach provided similar results 2 years after stent removal (88% vs. 90.9%, respectively) and similar treatment-related morbidity [79]. Short biliary strictures respond better to endoscopic therapy [80], and severe CP and long length stricture are predictors for stricture recurrence [81]. After 1 year of unsuccessful endoscopy therapy, surgery should be considered.

3.4.2 Pseudocyst and pancreatic duct leak

Approximately one-third of patients with CP develop pancreatic pseudocyst (PPC) during the course of their disease, and less than 10% of these cases will resolve spontaneously [82]. PPCs should be differentiated from cystic neoplasm.

The indications for PPC drainage are the presence of symptoms (abdominal pain, gastric obstruction, early satiety, weight loss, and jaundice), progressively cyst enlargement, or complications (infection, bleeding, rupture, and fistulization to adjacent hollow structures) [45, 83]. Asymptomatic pseudocysts can safely be kept under observation, provided they are carefully monitored and do not increase in size.

Endoscopic therapy of PPCs consists of transmural drainage (EUS-guided or conventional) with plastic or dedicated stents (PPCs ≥5 cm, no communication with pancreatic duct), endoscopic transpapillary drainage (PPC < 5 cm, communicating with pancreatic duct), or using a combination of these techniques [84]. Technical success is defined as insertion of the stent between the PPC and the digestive lumen [85]; instead clinical success is defined as disappearance of symptoms with resolution of the PPC or a decrease to less than 2 cm [86]. Compared with percutaneous drainage, endoscopic drainage is associated with higher clinical success rate, fewer reinterventions, shorter hospital stay, similar morbidity, and recurrence rate [87].

For an adequate treatment planning CT scan, MRI, EUS, and/or ERCP should be performed before PPC drainage to diagnose 1) the presence of necrotic debris inside the fluid collection (this may impede endoscopic drainage), 2) main pancreatic duct rupture (partial or complete), and 3) the presence of pseudoaneurysms close to the pseudocyst. If no ductal rupture is present, only transmural drainage can be performed; if partial ductal rupture is present, stent placement bridging the rupture is associated with the treatment success; if complete ductal rupture is present, long-term indwelling of transmural stents should be considered to avoid PPC recurrence [45, 88, 89]. Other technical aspects are underlined in Section 2.4.2.

3.4.3 Vascular complications

During CP progression, patients can develop, although rare, vascular complications that are difficult to treat and are responsible for significant morbidity and mortality. The CP-related vascular complications can be classified into arterial and venous (splanchnic thrombosis with splenic vein thrombosis) [90]. For the management of vascular complications, both surgical and nonsurgical interventions (endovascular, percutaneous, and endoscopic using EUS) are available. Nowadays, nonsurgical treatment options are the first-line therapy for these complications [90]. Obviously in this paragraph, we will focus on endoscopic technique.

Arterial complications are reported in 1.3–10% of patients with CP, and pseudoaneurysm is the most common arterial complications (approximately 70% of bleeding complications in CP, with a reported mortality rate of 15–50%) [91, 92]. They can be asymptomatic or present with hemorrhage due to rupture (hemosuccus pancreaticus, gastrointestinal bleeding, or intra-retroperitoneal hemorrhage), pain, or obstructive symptoms [92]. All pseudoaneurysms diagnosed on imaging require treatment irrespective of size as they have a high risk of rupture and life-threatening hemorrhage. The endoscopic approach is used for pseudoaneurysms detected on EUS. Hence, EUS-guided injection of the embolic agent (thrombin) is reserved for pseudoaneurysms arising from splenic and gastroduodenal arteries [90, 93].

The reported prevalence of venous thrombosis in patients with CP ranges from 3 to 41.7% with a pooled prevalence of 11.6%. Of the splanchnic veins, splenic vein thrombosis is the most common due to its proximity to the pancreas (prevalence ranging from 1.5 to 41.7%). Splenic vein thrombosis can extend to the portal vein in 1.5–4% of patients. Mesenteric venous thrombosis is uncommon and is reported in 0.8–1.1% of patients with CP [94]. In patients presenting with gastrointestinal variceal bleeding, endoscopic or surgical intervention of the gastroesophageal varices is required. Endoscopic therapy is preferred for patients without significant pancreatic symptoms as they do not require surgery for CP [90]. Esophageal varices can be treated either with banding or sclerotherapy with conventional sclerosants. For gastric or fundal varices, these are not effective, and recent studies have reported reasonable success rates with cyanoacrylate glue injection [95].

4. Conclusions

Endotherapy is not only limited either to the diagnosis of AP and CP or to the management of biliary/pancreatic duct stones and strictures but also associated with the treatment of AP and CP complications.

The technological growth of endoscopy has made enormous progress, allowing a less invasive treatment of these pathologies. Obviously, to have a safe role and correct timing, discussions on treatments must be taken by a multidisciplinary group.

Conflict of interest

The authors declare no conflict of interest.

Author details

Stefano Benvenuti, Eleonora Pinese* and Ilenia Barbuscio
Department of Gastroenterology and Endoscopic Unit, Ospedale Ca' Foncello, Treviso, Italy

*Address all correspondence to: eleonora.pinese@aulss2.veneto.it

References

[1] Spanier B, Dijkgraaf M, Bruno M. Epidemiology, aetiology and outcome of acute and chronic pancreatitis: An update. Best Practice & Research. Clinical Gastroenterology. 2008;**22**:45-63. DOI: 10.1097/01.sla.0000167761.70021.4d

[2] Zerem E. Treatment of severe acute pancreatitis and its complications. World Journal of Gastroenterology. 2014;**20**:13879-13892. DOI: 10.3748/wjg.v20.i38.13879

[3] Majumder S, Chari S. Chronic pancreatitis. The Lancet. 2016;**387**: 1957-1966. DOI: 10.1016/S0140-6736(16)00097-0

[4] Drewes A, Bouwense S, Campbell C, et al. Guidelines for the understanding and management of pain in chronic pancreatitis. Pancreatology. 2017;**17**:720-731. DOI: 10.1016/j.pan.2017.07.006

[5] Boxhoorn L, Voermans R, Bouwense S. Acute Pancreatitis. Lancet. 2020;**396**:726-734. DOI: 10.1016/S0140-6736(20)31310-6

[6] Anderson K, Brown L, Daniel P. Alanine transaminase rather than abdominal ultrasound alone is an important investigation to justify cholecystectomy in patients presenting with acute pancreatitis. HPB: The Official Journal of the International Hepato Pancreato Biliary Association. 2010;**12**:342-347. DOI: 10.1111/j.1477-2574.2010.00173.x

[7] Kotwal V, Talukdar R, Levy M. Role of endoscopic ultrasound during hospitalization for acute pancreatitis. World Journal of Gastroenterology. 2010;**16**:4888-4891. DOI: 10.3748/wjg.v16.i39.4888

[8] Zaheer A, Anwar M, Donohoe C. The diagnostic accuracy of endoscopic ultrasound in suspected biliary obstruction and its impact on endoscopic retrograde cholangiopancreatography burden in real clinical practice: A consecutive analysis. European Journal of Gastroenterology & Hepatology. 2013;**25**:850-857. DOI: 10.1097/MEG.0b013e32835ee5d0

[9] Buxbaum J, Abbas Fehmi S, Sultan S. ASGE guideline on the role of endoscopy in the evaluation and management of choledocholithiasis. Gastrointestinal Endoscopy. 2019;**89**:1075-1105.e15. DOI: 10.1016/j.gie.2018.10.001

[10] AGA Institute Governing Board. AGA institute medical position statement on acute pancreatitis. Gastroenterology. 2007;**132**:2019-2021. DOI: 10.1053/j.gastro.2007.03.066

[11] Kozu T, Suda K, Toki F. Pancreatic development and anatomical variation. Gastrointestinal Endoscopy Clinics of North America. 1995;**5**:1-30. DOI: doi.org/10.1016/S1052-5157(18)30458-6

[12] Bertin C, Pelletier A, Vullierme M, et al. Pancreas divisum is not a cause of pancreatitis by itself but acts as a partner of genetic mutations. The American journal of Gastroenterology. 2012;**107**:311-317. DOI: 10.1038/ajg.2011.424

[13] Manfredi R, Costamagna G, Brizi M, Spina S, Maresca G, Vecchioli A, et al. Pancreas divisum and "santorinicele": Diagnosis with dynamic MR cholangiopancreatography with secretin stimulation. Radiology. 2000;**217**:403-408. DOI: 10.1148/radiology.217.2.r00nv29403

[14] Chey W, Chang T. Secretin: Historical perspective and current status. Pancreas. 2014;**43**:162-182. DOI: 10.1097/01.mpa.0000437325.29728.d6

[15] Mariani A, Arcidiacono P, Curioni S, et al. Diagnostic yield of ERCP and secretin-enhanced MRCP and EUS in patients with acute recurrent pancreatitis of unknown aetiology. Digestive and Liver Disease. 2009;**41**:753-758. DOI: 10.1016/j.dld.2009.01.009

[16] Gutta A, Fogel E, Sherman E. Identification and Management of Pancreas Divisum. Expert Review of Gastroenterology & Hepatology. 2019;**13**:1089-1105. DOI: 10.1080/17474124.2019.1685871

[17] Sugiyama M, Atomi Y, Kuroda A. Pancreatic disorders associated with anomalous pancreaticobiliary junction. Surgery. 1999;**126**:492-497. DOI: doi.org/10.1016/S0039-6060(99)70090-5

[18] Kamisawa T, Egawa N, Tsuruta K, Okamoto A, Mtsukawa M. Pancreatitis associated with congenital abnormalities of the pancreaticobiliary system. Hepato-Gastroenterology. 2005;**52**:223-229

[19] Elton E, Hanson B, Biber B, Howell D. Dilated common channel syndrome: Endoscopic diagnosis, treatment, and relationship to choledochocele formation. Gastrointestinal Endoscopy. 1998;**47**:471-478. DOI: 10.1016/S0016-5107(98)70247-0

[20] Working Group IAPAPAAPG. IAP/APA evidence-based guidelines for the management of acute pancreatitis. Pancreatology. 2013;**13**:e1-e15. DOI: 10.1016/j.pan.2013.07.063

[21] Nesvaderani M, Eslick G, Vagg D, et al. Epidemiology, aetiology and outcomes of acute pancreatitis: s retrospective cohort study. International Journal of Surgery. 2015;**23**:68-74. DOI: doi.org/10.1016/j.ijsu.2015.07.701

[22] Smith I, Ramesh J, Kyanam Kabir Baig K, et al. Emerging role of endoscopic ultrasound in the diagnostic evaluation of idiopathic pancreatitis. The American Journal of the Medical Sciences. 2015;**350**:229-234. DOI: 10.1097/MAJ.0000000000000541

[23] Lehman G. Endoscopic sphincter of Oddi manometry: A clinical practice and research tool. Gastrointestinal Endoscopy. 1991;**37**:490-492. DOI: 10.1016/s0016-5107(91)70792-x

[24] Afghani E, Lo S, Covington P, Cash B, Pandol S. Sphincter of Oddi function and risk factors for dysfunction. Frontiers in Nutrition. 2017;**4**:1. DOI: 10.3389/fnut.2017.00001

[25] Banks P, Bollen T, Dervenis C. Classification of acute pancreatitis - 2012: Revision of the Atlanta classification and definitions by international consensus. Gut. 2013;**62**:102-111. DOI: 10.1136/gutjnl-2012-302779

[26] Manrai M, Kochhar R, Gupta V. Outcome of acute pancreatic and Peripancreatic collections occurring in patients with acute pancreatitis. Annals of Surgery. 2018;**267**:357-363. DOI: 10.1097/SLA.0000000000002065

[27] Banks P, Freeman M. Practice guidelines in acute pancreatitis. The American Journal of Gastroenterology. 2006;**101**:2379-2400. DOI: 10.1111/j.1572-0241.2006.00856.x

[28] Andrén-Sandberg A, Dervenis C. Pancreatic pseudocysts in the 21st century. Part II: Natural history. Journal of the Pancreas: JOP. 2004;**5**:64-70

[29] Kahaleh M, Shami V, Conaway M. Endoscopic ultrasound drainage of pancreatic pseudocyst: A prospective comparison with conventional endoscopic drainage. Endoscopy. 2006;**38**:335-359. DOI: 10.1055/s-2006-925249

[30] Baron T, Harewood G, Morgan D, Yates M. Outcome differences after endoscopic drainage of pancreatic necrosis, acute pancreatic pseudocysts, and chronic pancreatic pseudocysts. Gastrointestinal Endoscopy. 2002;**56**: 7-17. DOI: 10.1067/mge.2002.125106

[31] Bapaye A, Itoi T, Kongkam P, Dubale N, Mukai S. New fully covered large-bore wide-flare removable metal stent for drainage of pancreatic fluid collections: Results of a multicenter study. Digestive Endoscopy. 2015;**27**: 499-504. DOI: 10.1111/den.12421

[32] Itoi T, Binmoeller K, Shah J, et al. Clinical evaluation of a novel lumen-apposing metal stent for endosonography-guided pancreatic pseudocyst and gallbladder drainage. Gastrointestinal Endoscopy. 2012;**75**:870-876. DOI: 10.1016/j.gie.2011.10.020

[33] Lang G, Fritz C, Bhat T. EUS-guided drainage of peripancreatic fluid collections with lumen-apposing metal stents and plastic double-pigtail stents: Comparison of efficacy and adverse event rates. Gastrointestinal Endoscopy. 2018;**87**:150-157. DOI: 10.1016/j.gie.2017.06.029

[34] Bang J, Navaneethen U, Hasan M, Sutton B, Hawes R, Varadarajulu S. Non-superiority of lumen-apposing metal stents over plastic stents for drainage of walled-off necrosis in a randomised trial. Gut. 2019;**68**:1200-1209. DOI: doi.org/10.1136/gutjnl-2017-315335

[35] Boxhoorn L, Timmerhuis H, Verdonk R. Diagnosis and treatment of pancreatic duct disruption or disconnection: An international expert survey and casevignette study. HPB: The Official Journal of the International Hepato Pancreato Biliary Association. 2021;**23**:1201-1208. DOI: 10.1016/j.hpb.2020.11.1148

[36] Bang J, Wilcox C, Navaneethan U, Hasan M, Peter S, Christein J, et al. Impact of disconnected pancreatic duct syndrome on the endoscopic Management of Pancreatic Fluid Collections. Annals of Surgery. 2018;**267**:561-568. DOI: 10.1097/SLA.0000000000002082

[37] Verma S, Rana S. Disconnected pancreatic duct syndrome: Updated review on clinical implications and management. Pancreatology. 2020;**20**:1035-1044. DOI: 10.1016/j.pan.2020.07.402

[38] Whitcomb D, Shimosegava T, Chari S. International consensus statements on early chronic pancreatitis. Recommendations from the working Group for the International Consensus Guidelines for chronic pancreatitis in collaboration with the International Association of Pancreatology. Pancreatology. 2018;**18**:516-527. DOI: 10.1016/j.pan.2018.05.008

[39] Issa Y, Kempeneers M, Santvoort H. Diagnostic performance of imaging modalities in chronic pancreatitis: A systematic review and meta-analysis. European Radiology. 2017;**27**:3820-3844. DOI: 10.1007/s00330-016-4720-9

[40] Löhr J, Dominguez-Munoz E, Rosendahl J. United European gastroenterology evidence-based guidelines for the diagnosis and therapy of chronic pancreatitis (HaPanEU). United European Gastroenterology Journal. 2017;**5**:153-199. DOI: 10.1177/2050640616684695

[41] Raimondo M, Wallace M. Diagnosis of early chronic pancreatitis by endoscopic ultrasound. Are we there yet? Journal of the Pancreas: JOP. 2004;**5**:1-7

[42] Catalano M, Sahai A, Levy M. EUS-based criteria for the diagnosis of chronic pancreatitis: The Rosemont classification. Gastrointestinal Endoscopy. 2009;**69**: 1251-1261. DOI: 10.1016/j.gie.2008.07.043

[43] Sarles H, Camarena J, Gomez-Santana C. Radiolucent and calcified pancreatic lithiasis: Two different diseases. Role of alcohol and heredity. Scandinavian Journal of Gastroenterology. 1992;**27**:71-76. DOI: 10.3109/00365529209011170

[44] Frulloni L, Gabbrielli A, Pezzilli R, et al. Chronic pancreatitis: Report from a multicenter Italian survey (PanCroInfAISP) on 893 patients. Digestive and Liver Disease. 2009;**41**:311-317. DOI: 10.1016/j.dld.2008.07.316

[45] Dumonceau J, Delhaye M, Tringali A, et al. Endoscopic treatment of chronic pancreatitis: European Society of Gastrointestinal Endoscopy (ESGE) guideline - updated august 2018. Endoscopy. 2019;**51**:179-193. DOI: doi.org/10.1055/a-0822-0832

[46] Sharzehi K. Management of pancreatic duct stones. Current Gastroenterology Reports. 2019;**21**:63. DOI: 10.1007/s11894-019-0727-0

[47] Tandan M, Nageshwar R. Endotherapy in chronic pancreatitis. World Journal of Gastroenterology. 2013;**19**:6156-6164. DOI: 10.3748/wjg.v19.i37.6156

[48] Farnbacher M, Schoen C, Rabenstein T. Pancreatic duct stones in chronic pancreatitis: Criteria for treatment intensity and success. Gastrointestinal Endoscopy. 2002;**56**: 501-506. DOI: 10.1067/mge.2002.128162

[49] Inui K, Masamune A, Igarashi Y, et al. Management of pancreatolithiasis: A nationwide survey in Japan. Pancreas. 2018;**47**:708-714. DOI: 10.1097/MPA.0000000000001071

[50] Tandan M, Reddy D, Santosh D, et al. Extracorporeal shock wave lithotripsy and endotherapy for pancreatic calculi-a large single center experience. Indian Journal of Gastroenterology. 2010;**29**:143-148. DOI: 10.1007/s12664-010-0035-y

[51] Moole H, Jaeger A, Bechtold M, et al. Success of extracorporeal shockwave lithotripsy in chronic calcific pancreatitis management: A meta-analysis and systematic review. Pancreas. 2016;**45**:651-658. DOI: 10.1097/MPA.0000000000000512

[52] Li B, Liao Z, Du T, et al. Risk factors for complications of pancreatic extracorporeal shock wave lithotripsy. Endoscopy. 2014;**46**:1092-1100. DOI: 10.1055/s-0034-1377753

[53] Dumonceau J, Costamagna G, Tringali A, et al. Treatment for painful calcified chronic pancreatitis: Extracorporeal shock wave lithotripsy versus endoscopic treatment: A randomised controlled trial. Gut. 2007;**56**:545-552. DOI: 10.1136/gut.2006.096883

[54] Vaysse T, Boytchev I, Antoni G, et al. Efficacy and safety of extracorporeal shock wave lithotripsy for chronic pancreatitis. Scandinavian Journal of Gastroenterology. 2016;**51**:1380-1385. DOI: doi.org/10.1080/00365521.2016.1209688

[55] McCarty T, Sobani Z, Rustagi T. Per-oral pancreatoscopy with intraductal lithotripsy for difficult pancreatic duct stones: A systematic review and meta-analysis. Endoscopy International Open.

2020;**8**:E1460-E1470. DOI: 10.1055/a-1236-3187

[56] Saghir S, Mashiana H, Mohan B, et al. Efficacy of pancreatoscopy for pancreatic duct stones: A systematic review and meta-analysis. World Journal of Gastroenterology. 2020;**26**:5207-5219. DOI: 10.3748/wjg.v26.i34.5207

[57] Han S, Shah R, Brauer B, et al. A comparison of endoscopic retrograde pancreatography with or without pancreatoscopy for removal of pancreatic duct stones. Pancreas. 2019;**48**:690-697. DOI: 10.1097/MPA.0000000000001317

[58] Cremer M, Devière J, Delhaye M, et al. Stenting in severe chronic pancreatitis: Results of medium-term follow-up in seventy-six patients. Endoscopy. 1991;**23**:171-176. DOI: 10.1055/s-2007-1010649

[59] Delhaye M, Matos C, Devière J. Endoscopic management of chronic pancreatitis. Gastrointestinal Endoscopy Clinics of North America. 2003;**13**:717-742. DOI: doi.org/10.1016/S1052-5157(03)00070-9

[60] Kirkegård J, Mortensen F, Cronin-Fenton D. Chronic pancreatitis and pancreatic cancer risk: A systematic review and meta-analysis. The American Journal of Gastroenterology. 2017;**112**:1366-1372. DOI: 10.1038/ajg.2017.218

[61] Binmoller K, Rathod V, Soehendra N. Endoscopic therapy of pancreatic strictures. Gastrointestinal Endoscopy Clinics of North America. 1998;**8**:125-142

[62] Kwon CI, Gromski M, Sherman S, et al. Clinical response to dorsal duct drainage via the minor papilla in refractory obstructing chronic calcific pancreatitis. Endoscopy. 2017;**49**:371-377. DOI: 10.1055/s-0042-120996

[63] Cahen D, Gouma D, Nyo Y, et al. Endoscopic versus surgical drainage of the pancreatic duct in chronic pancreatitis. The New England Journal of Medicine. 2007;**356**:676-684. DOI: 10.1056/NEJMoa060610

[64] Dalhaye M, Arvanitakis M, Verset G, Cremer M, Deviere J. Long-term clinical outcome after endoscopic pancreatic ductal drainage for patients with painful chronic pancreatitis. Gastroenterología y Hepatología. 2004;**2**:1096-1106. DOI: doi.org/10.1016/S1542-3565(04)00544-0

[65] Costamagna G, Bulajic M, Tringali A, et al. Multiple stenting of refractory pancreatic duct strictures in severe chronic pancreatitis: Long-term results. Endoscopy. 2006;**38**:254-259. DOI: 10.1055/s-2005-921069

[66] Tringali A, Bove V, Vadalà di Prampero SF, et al. Long-term follow-up after multiple plastic stenting for refractory pancreatic duct strictures in chronic pancreatitis. Endoscopy. 2019;**51**:930-935. DOI: 10.1055/a-0959-6163

[67] Matsubara S, Sasahira N, Isayama H, et al. Prospective pilot study of fully covered self-expandable metal stents for refractory benign pancreatic duct strictures: Long-term outcomes. Endoscopy International Open. 2016;**4**:E1215-E1222. DOI: 10.1055/s-0042-115934

[68] Tringali A, Vadalà di Prampero SF, Landi R, et al. Fully covered self-expandable metal stents to dilate persistent pancreatic strictures in chronic pancreatitis: Long-term follow-up from a prospective study. Gastrointestinal Endoscopy. 2018;**88**:939-946. DOI: 10.1016/j.gie.2018.08.019

[69] Shen Y, Liu M, Chen M, Li Y, Lu Y, Zou X. Covered metal stent or multiple

plastic stents for refractory pancreatic ductal strictures in chronic pancreatitis: A systematic review. Pancreatology. 2014;**14**:87-90. DOI: 10.1016/j.pan.2013.12.005

[70] Sharaiha R, Novikov A, Weaver K, et al. Fully covered self- expanding metal stents for refractory pancreatic duct strictures in symptomatic chronic pancreatitis, US experience. Endoscopy International Open. 2019;**7**:E1419-E1423. DOI: 10.1055/a-0858-2169

[71] Nguyen-Tang T, Dumonceau J. Endoscopic treatment in chronic pancreatitis, timing, duration and type of intervention. Best Practice & Research. Clinical Gastroenterology. 2010;**24**:281-298. DOI: doi.org/10.1016/j.bpg.2010.03.002

[72] Devière J. EUS-guided pancreatic duct drainage: A rare indication in need of prospective evidence. Gastrointestinal Endoscopy. 2017;**85**:178-180. DOI: 10.1016/j.gie.2016.08.041

[73] Kahaleh M, Hernandez A, Tokar J, et al. EUS-guided pancreaticogastrostomy: Analysis of its efficacy to drain inaccessible pancreatic ducts. Gastrointestinal Endoscopy. 2007;**65**:224-230. DOI: doi.org/10.1016/j.gie.2006.05.008

[74] Hu B, Sun B, Cai Q, et al. Asia-Pacific consensus guidelines for endoscopic management of benign biliary strictures. Gastrointestinal Endoscopy. 2017;**86**:44-58. DOI: 10.1016/j.gie.2017.02.031

[75] Abdallah A, Krige J, Bornman P. Biliary tract obstruction in chronic pancreatitis. HPB: The Official Journal of the International Hepato Pancreato Biliary Association. 2007;**9**:421-428. DOI: 10.1080/13651820701774883

[76] Craig P. Role of endoscopic stenting for biliary strictures in chronic pancreatitis. Digestive Endoscopy. 2012;**24**(Suppl. 1):38-42. DOI: doi.org/10.1111/j.1443-1661.2012.01283.x

[77] Dumonceau J, Tringali A, Papanikolaou I, et al. Endoscopic biliary stenting: Indications, choice of stents, and results: European Society of Gastrointestinal Endoscopy (ESGE) clinical guideline – Updated October 2017. Endoscopy. 2018;**50**:910-930. DOI: doi.org/10.1055/a-0659-9864

[78] Siriwardana H, Siriwardena A. Systematic appraisal of the role of metallic endobiliary stents in the treatment of benign bile duct stricture. Annals of Surgery. 2005;**242**:10-19. DOI: 10.1097/01.sla.0000167761.70021.4d

[79] Haapamäki C, Kylänpää L, Udd M, et al. Randomized multicenter study of multiple plastic stents vs. covered self-expandable metallic stent in the treatment of biliary stricture in chronic pancreatitis. Endoscopy. 2015;**47**:605-610. DOI: 10.1055/s-0034-1391331

[80] Ohyama H, Mikata R, Ishihara T, et al. Efficacy of multiple biliary stenting for refractory benign biliary strictures due to chronic calcifying pancreatitis. World Journal of Gastrointestinal Endoscopy. 2017;**9**:12-18. DOI: 10.4253/wjge.v9.i1.12

[81] Lakhtakia S, Reddy N, Dolak W, et al. Long-term outcomes after temporary placement of a self-expanding fully covered metal stent for benign biliary strictures secondary to chronic pancreatitis. Gastrointestinal Endoscopy. 2020;**91**:361-9.e3. DOI: 10.1016/j.gie.2019.08.037

[82] Beckingham I, Krige J, Bornman P, et al. Endoscopic management of pancreatic pseudocysts. British Journal of Surgery. 1997;**84**:1638-1645. DOI: 10.1046/j.1365-2168.1997.00561.x

[83] Law R, Baron T. Endoscopic management of pancreatic pseudocysts and necrosis. Expert Review of Gastroenterology & Hepatology. 2015;**9**:167-175. DOI: 10.1586/17474124.2014.943186

[84] Barthet M, Lamblin G, Gasmi M, et al. Clinical usefulness of a treatment algorithm for pancreatic pseudocysts. Gastrointestinal Endoscopy. 2008;**67**:245-252. DOI: 10.1016/j.gie.2007.06.014

[85] Shah R, Shah J, Waxman I, et al. Safety and efficacy of endoscopic ultrasound-guided drainage of pancreatic fluid collections with lumen-apposing covered self-expanding metal stents. Clinical Gastroenterology and Hepatology. 2015;**13**:747-738. DOI: 10.1016/j.cgh.2014.09.047

[86] Yoon S, Lee I, Choi M. Metal versus plastic stents for drainage of pancreatic fluid collection: A meta-analysis. United European Gastroenterology Journal. 2018;**6**:729-738. DOI: 10.1177/2050640618761702

[87] Khan M, Hammad T, Khan Z, et al. Endoscopic versus percutaneous management for symptomatic pancreatic fluid collections: A systematic review and meta-analysis. Endoscopy International Open. 2018;**06**:E474-E483. DOI: 10.1055/s-0044-102299

[88] Bang J, Wilcox C, Trevino J, et al. Factors impacting treatment outcomes in the endoscopic management of walled-off pancreatic necrosis. Journal of Gastroenterology and Hepatology. 2013;**28**:1725-1732. DOI: 10.1111/jgh.12328

[89] Arvanitakis M, Delhaye M, Bali M, et al. Pancreatic-fluid collections: A randomized controlled trial regarding stent removal after endoscopic transmural drainage. Gastrointestinal Endoscopy. 2007;**65**:609-619. DOI: 10.1016/j.gie.2006.06.083

[90] Agarwal A, Kalayarason R, Javed A. Vascular complications in chronic pancreatitis. In: Dominguez-Munõz JE, editor. Clinical Pancreatology for Practising Gastroenterologists and Surgeons. Second ed. Chichester: Wiley; 2021. pp. 322-332. DOI: 10.1002/9781119570097.ch41

[91] Verde F, Fishman E, Johnson P. Arterial pseudoaneurysms complicating pancreatitis: Literature review. Journal of Computer Assisted Tomography. 2015;**39**:7-12. DOI: 10.1097/RCT.0000000000000153

[92] Chiang K, Chen T, Hsu J. Management of chronic pancreatitis complicated with a bleeding pseudoaneurysm. World Journal of Gastroenterology. 2014;**20**:16132-16137. DOI: 10.3748/wjg.v20.i43.16132

[93] Gamanagatti S, Thingujam U, Garg P, et al. Endoscopic ultrasound guided thrombin injection of angiographically occult pancreatitis associated visceral artery pseudoaneurysms: Case series. World Journal of Gastrointestinal Endoscopy. 2015;7:1107-1113. DOI: 10.4253/wjge.v7.i13.1107

[94] Xu W, Qi X, Chen J et al. Prevalence of splanchnic vein thrombosis in pancreatitis: A systematic review and meta-analysis of observational studies. Gastroenterology Research and Practice 2015;**2015**:1-23. DOI: doi.org/10.1155/2015/245460

[95] Al-Osaimi A, Cadwell S. Medical and endoscopic management of gastric varices. Seminars in Interventional Radiology. 2011;**28**:273-282. DOI: 10.1055/s-0031-1284453

Chapter 5

ERCP and EUS in Management of Pancreatitis

Michael Okello and Derick Kayondo

Abstract

Interventional endoscopic procedures like Endoscopic Retrograde Cholangiopancreatography (ERCP) and endoscopic ultrasound (EUS) have a major role in the minimally invasive management of acute and chronic pancreatitis and their complications. These complications may be due to pancreaticolithiasis, main pancreatic duct strictures, trauma, infections, autoimmune pancreatitis and pancreatic neoplasms. ERCP and endoscopic ultrasound scan are important as both diagnostic and therapeutic interventions. The commonly managed complications by ERCP and EUS include; pancreatic duct stones, main pancreatic duct strictures, pancreatic pseudocysts and pancreatic walled off necrosis. These endoscopic interventions have the advantage of cosmesis, short hospital stay and can be safely used even in very sick, critical or elderly patients without necessarily increasing the morbidity and mortality associated with open surgical approaches.

Keywords: ERCP, endoscopic ultrasound scan, pancreatitis, pancreatic strictures, stones, neoplasms

1. Introduction

Endoscopic Retrograde Cholangiopancreatography (ERCP) has been employed in the diagnosis and management of biliary tract and pancreatic diseases over the years with the first diagnostic ERCP performed in 1968 by McCune and colleagues [1]. With the presence of less invasive diagnostic procedures such as Contrast enhanced Computed Tomography (CT), abdominal ultrasound, Endoscopic Ultrasound (EUS), Magnetic Resonance Cholangiopancreatography (MRCP) and better blood biomarkers, the popularity of ERCP as a diagnostic procedure has reduced overtime due to the ERCP-associated complications such as pancreatitis, bleeding which negatively impact its relevance as a routine diagnostic tool in pancreatic and bile duct pathologies. Preference has now shifted to the less risky non-invasive diagnostic procedures that involve no duct instrumentation.

The most common causes of acute pancreatitis are gallstones (40–70%) and alcohol (25–35%) [2]. ERCP is mainly utilized in management of gall stone pancreatitis especially among patients with cholangitis, biliary obstruction and pancreatic duct disruption. ERCP also has wide applications in the diagnosis of ductal changes in chronic pancreatitis with application of EUS in diagnosis of the parenchymal changes and intraductal stones with high accuracy. ERCP and EUS also have roles in diagnosis and management of various acute, subacute and chronic pancreatitis etiologies (such as intraductal gall stones, sphincter of Oddi dysfunction) and complications (such as pancreatic duct leaks, pancreatic pseudocysts) among others.

The potential benefits must be weighed against the associated risks of complications when selecting patients to undergo ERCP or its different therapeutic interventions.

2. Timing and role of ERCP in acute biliary pancreatitis

Acute biliary pancreatitis results from transient obstruction of the common bile duct by stones. Majority of the stones spontaneously pass into the duodenum followed by resolution of the acute pancreatitis [2]. In a few of the patients, persistent choledocholithiasis can lead to pancreatic duct and/or biliary tree obstruction resulting into severe/persistent pancreatitis and/or cholangitis with resolution and complication risk reduction on removal of the offending stones [3].

Stone can be extracted during ERCP by either balloon catheters or dormia stone extraction baskets after either endoscopic sphincterotomy (papillotomy) and/or endoscopic papillary balloon dilatation (sphincteroplasty). Papillary balloon dilatation is however not routinely recommended due to a lower technical success for stone clearance and a presumed increased risk of pancreatitis. It can however be considered in patients with coagulopathies or altered anatomy with smaller (<8 mm) stones [4]. Endoscopic sphincterotomy with stone extraction is associated with 80–90% success rate in common bile duct (CBD) stones treatment. In cases of irretrievable biliary stones, temporary biliary plastic or metallic stents can be placed to relieve the obstruction followed by a second attempt at stone removal combined with either mechanical or extracorporeal shock wave lithotripsy (ESWL). Failure of ERCP, EUS mechanical or ESWL ultimately means surgical intervention which can be open or laparoscopic cholecystectomy with choledocholithotomy to remove the CBD stones done during CBD exploration. For cases of ERCP with stenting, the stents may however, be associated with complications such as cholangitis and so should be removed or exchanged every 3–6 months. Definitive stenting is recommended in the elderly with a limited life expectancy and co-morbidities with caution due to the high rates of complications such as cholangitis with associated high mortality [4].

There is consensus among different meta-analyses and guidelines on the role and timing of early ERCP with endoscopic sphincterotomy (ES) in case of acute biliary pancreatitis in the presence of cholangitis and/or persistent cholestasis. However there is obvious lack of agreement on the role and timing of ERCP in mild or severe predicted acute biliary pancreatitis in the absence of cholangitis or persistent cholestasis [5]. Neoptolemus J.P. et al. [6] conducted a randomized controlled trial involving 121 patients with suspected biliary acute pancreatitis using the modified Glasgow system for severity stratification. Early ERCP done within 72 hours plus Endoscopic sphincterotomy for those with common bile duct stones was associated with reduction in complications and shorter hospital stay significantly among those with severe acute pancreatitis when compared with those on conventional treatment. The reduction in complications was still noticed even after excluding those with associated cholangitis. However, no difference in mortality was noted. Another randomized control trial by Fan S T et al. [7] randomized 195 patients with acute pancreatitis to two arms, either early ERCP done within 24 hours after admission with endoscopic papillotomy for ampullary and common bile duct stones or conservative treatment and selective ERCP with or without endoscopic papillotomy in those that deteriorated. Early ERCP with/without endoscopic papillotomy was associated with reduction in biliary sepsis in both patients with mild or severe acute pancreatitis with no major differences in incidence of local or systemic complications between the two groups. The mortality rate was however lower in the early ERCP with or without endoscopic papillotomy group [7]. Another study by Folsch et al. [8] demonstrated no reduction in complications or mortality with early ERCP within 72 hours among patients with acute biliary pancreatitis with no obstruction. This study suggests that early ERCP is only beneficial among patients with acute pancreatitis complicated by acute cholangitis and biliary tree obstruction, and not in severe acute pancreatitis complicated in the absence of the above complications.

Based on meta-analysis, early ERCP with sphincterotomy (within 24–72 hours) had an overall significant reduction in complication rate among patients with biliary pancreatitis (41.8% versus 31.3%, P = 0.03, k = 3) significantly among those with severe disease (57.1% versus 18.2%, P = 0.0001, k = 2) with no overall significant effect on the mortality rate (7.2% versus 6.4%, P = 0.46, k = 3) [9]. Similar findings were noted in a meta-analysis by Moretti et al. when comparing early ERCP vs. conservative management in acute biliary pancreatitis. Early ERCP was associated with reduction in complications and mortality rates by 31% and 6% respectively with significant reduction in complication rates among patients with severe pancreatitis compared to mild pancreatitis (pooled rate difference of 38.5% vs. 1.8%) [10].

ERCP should not be routinely performed in patients with acute biliary pancreatitis due to its invasiveness and risk for complications. Early ERCP has been demonstrated to reduce complication rates among patients with severe acute biliary pancreatitis in the absence of cholangitis or biliary obstruction unlike among patients with mild disease. Early ERCP +ES may be considered among patients with acute biliary pancreatitis with severe biliary pancreatitis rather than among patients with mild acute biliary pancreatitis unless when having standard indications for ERCP + ES such as cholangitis, biliary obstruction [11]. However, proponents of early conservative management argue that early routine ERCP may lead to unnecessary ERCPs with related complications as the offending gallstone has passed in majority of the cases at the time of diagnosis [12, 13] and also with looming uncertainty of whether early ERCP improved prognosis of acute gallstone pancreatitis. Early ERCP is also technically difficult in acute pancreatitis due to ampulla and duodenal edema. It is therefore recommended by the ESGE that ERCP with or without endoscopic sphincterotomy among patients with acute biliary pancreatitis without cholangitis be reserved for patients with persistent biliary obstruction after a period of conservative management regardless of the severity [14, 15]. Cholecystectomy can be performed later after ERCP + ES (usually 4 to 6 weeks) to prevent recurrence of the acute pancreatitis [9]. Among patients with mild acute biliary pancreatitis, early laparoscopic cholecystectomy with intraoperative cholangiography is recommended. If intraoperative cholangiography reveals common bile duct stones with failed laparoscopic clearance of the stones, then post-operative ERCP should be performed [9].

Less invasive imaging modalities such as EUS and MRCP should be used to screen for choledocholithiasis in suspicious cases in the absence of cholangitis and/or jaundice.

3. Microlithiasis

Microlithiasis/biliary sludge is a controversial etiology for acute pancreatitis. Biliary sludge is detected in 75% of the patients with recurrent idiopathic acute pancreatitis [16, 17]. Abdominal ultrasound has low sensitivity in diagnosis of biliary sludge. Bile analysis with microscopic examination for cholesterol crystals is the gold standard for diagnosing biliary sludge with however a sensitivity of 66% [18].

The bile for analysis can be obtained directly through common bile duct aspiration at ERCP or by duodenal aspiration of bile after cholecystokinin stimulation. EUS can also be utilized in diagnosis of microlithiasis/biliary sludge with a higher sensitivity and also applicability in evaluating other causes of idiopathic acute pancreatitis [18]. ERCP should be done 4–6 weeks after the initial presentation when the pancreatitis has resolved and if microlithiasis is detected, cholecystectomy or biliary sphincterotomy can be considered as management options depending on the patient's surgical risk [19].

4. Sphincter of Oddi dysfunction

Sphincter of Oddi Dysfunction (SOD) is the most frequent cause of idiopathic recurrent acute pancreatitis with a prevalence rate between 15–72% among patients with idiopathic recurrent pancreatitis using ERCP with raised SOD basal pressures at sphincter of Oddi manometry (SOM) as the gold standard for diagnosis and 50–87% among those with chronic pancreatitis [18, 20]. The pathogenesis of pancreatitis in SOD involves increase in the intrapancreatic ductal pressures. The elevation in the intraductal pressure results from either anatomic obstruction of the Sphincter of Oddi by fibrosis and/or inflammation or from functional obstruction caused by sphincter muscle spasms.

Endoscopic therapies such as pancreatic and biliary sphincterotomy can be employed in treating pancreas divisum and/or sphincter of Oddi dysfunction especially in patients with recurrent acute pancreatitis. These therapies are however associated with a significant risk of precipitating acute pancreatitis and hemorrhage, and so should be performed in specialized units and with careful patient selection [3, 21].

Endoscopic injection of botulinum toxin decreases pancreatitis episodes in 80% of patients with acute idiopathic pancreatitis. However, the effect is short-lived with also concerns regarding side effects. Dual sphincterotomy has been demonstrated to have lower rates of pancreatitis recurrence compared to either biliary or pancreatitic sphincterotomy alone.

Temporary pancreatic stent placement is recommended to prevent post-procedure pancreatitis [19, 21].

5. Pancreas divisum

Pancreas divisum (PD) is the most common anatomical variant of the pancreatic duct with an incidence of approximately 10% in the general population and symptomatic in only 5% of the patients [22]. PD has been shown to be a predisposing factor for chronic and recurrent pancreatitis and an incidental finding in idiopathic pancreatitis. However, its exact etiological role in pancreatitis is not well understood and still under study [23].

Contrast-enhanced CT and contrast-enhanced MRCP can be used in the diagnosis of PD with improved sensitivities with secretin provocation for better visualization of the ducts.

Endoscopic Ultrasound (EUS) has also been reported to have a high diagnostic accuracy for PD with a sensitivity of 87–95% with secretin enhancement (S-EUS) offering marginal benefit. Absence of a "stack sign" and the presence of a "crossed duct sign" are considered to be indicative of PD. ERCP is seldom used if no therapeutic interventions are intended due to the associated risks [23].

Therapeutic interventions are reserved for patients with recurrent attacks of acute pancreatitis, incases of a single episode of severe pancreatitis in the absence of any other identifiable etiology or in chronic pancreatitis with a modifiable target such as a stone, dilated dorsal duct or stricture [23]. Endoscopic and surgical therapies can be employed on the management of PD. Endoscopic therapy includes minor papilla endoscopic sphincterotomy, minor papilla orifice balloon dilatation and trans minor papilla dorsal duct stenting.

Papillary endotherapy is associated with an increased risk of post-procedural pancreatitis and therefore prophylactic temporary pancreatic stenting is recommended in addition to peri-procedural non-steroidal anti-inflammatory drugs (NSAIDs) are recommended to reduce the risk. Long-term dorsal pancreatic duct stenting though effective, is associated with possible complications such as occlusion, ductal perforation, acute pancreatitis and proximal or distal stent migration.

Surgical therapy includes surgical minor papilla sphincterotomy or surgical minor papilla sphincteroplasty.

For both endoscopic and surgical therapies, the response rate to therapy is higher in the recurrent pancreatitis group compared to chronic pancreatitis and the chronic pancreatic-type abdominal pain (76–80% Vs 42%- 69% Vs 33–54% with endotherapy and 83% Vs 67% Vs 52% with surgical therapy) [23]. Due to comparable response rates with both endoscopic and surgical therapies, endoscopic therapy is recommended as first line due to a more favorable complication and mortality rate. Surgery is preserved for patients with failed minor papilla cannulation, endotherapy or have altered anatomy such as Bilroth II anatomy [23].

6. Pancreatic and biliary tumors

Pancreatic and biliary tree tumors may present with acute or chronic pancreatitis due to obstruction of the pancreatic duct.

ERCP and EUS have applications in the diagnosis and management of ampullary tumors and intraductal papillary mucinous tumors of the pancreas. ERCP can help with visualization and biopsy sample collection from tumors involving the ampulla and periampullary region. EUS also can be utilized in evaluation of pancreatic and biliary tree masses causing pancreatitis and ultrasound-guided sample collection. Curative or palliative interventions such as endoscopic snare ampullectomy or ablative therapy can also be performed endoscopically. Recurrent pancreatitis for example in intraductal papillary mucinous tumors can be minimized by sphincterotomy with stenting.

7. Pancreatic duct leaks and pancreatic fluid collections

Pancreatic duct disruptions occur in both acute and chronic pancreatitis and in some cases in case of pancreatic trauma. Pancreatic duct leaks can complicate acute pancreatitis as a result of ductal epithelial disruptions by the inflammatory process and in chronic pancreatitis, as a result of ductal obstruction from inflammatory strictures and intraductal stones [24]. Pancreatic duct leaks may have variable presentations such as pancreatic fluid collections e.g. pseudocysts, pancreatic ascites, external pancreatic fistulas, disconnected duct syndrome among others. Pancreatic fluid collections may also result as a complication of pancreatic necrosis.

Diagnosis may be made using cross-sectional imaging studies such as Computed Tomograpgy (CT), secretin-enhanced MRCP or ultrasonography. Due to the associated risk of causing or worsening pancreatitis, ERCP is not employed for primary diagnostic purposes but rather for therapeutic interventions. EUS-guided Fine Needle Aspiration can be used to obtain pancreatic pseudocyst fluid for analysis for amylase levels, carcino-embryonic antigen (CEA) and cytology to differentiate pseudocyst from cystic neoplasms [24].

Pancreatic duct leaks may be effectively managed by endoscopic trans-papillary pancreatic duct stenting with a stent that bridges the leak diverting pancreatic fluid drainage from the ductal disruption to the duodenum.

Pancreatic pseudocysts occur as complications of acute or chronic pancreatitis and are usually asymptomatic except in a few cases. Pseudocysts and other pancreatic fluid collections can be managed endoscopically with a success rate of 70–97% [23, 25] and complication rate of 5–19% with complications such as hemorrhage and recurrence [26].

Endoscopic transluminal or trans-papillary drainage options with or without ultrasound are effective in draining these cysts and are usually performed 4 to 6 weeks after the acute pancreatitis episode resolves [23, 24]. Pancreatic pseudocysts can be drained via endoscopically created cysto-gastrostomies or cysto-enterostomies with subsequent stent placement. EUS is helpful in identification and preventing trauma to blood vessels during the procedure and also in situations where there is no visible bulge from the cyst in the gastrointestinal lumen. Though less popular recently, pancreatic fluid collections can also be managed with transmural or trans-papillary placement of plastic stents [25].

8. Pancreatic strictures

Pancreatic strictures can be diagnosed radiologically by CT and MRI/MRCP with supplementation with Endoscopic Ultrasound, secretin-enhanced MRCP, pancreatic function tests especially in the early stages with limited structural changes [27]. ESGE recommends treating painful dominant main pancreatic duct (MPD) strictures with insertion of a single stent across the dominant MPD stricture for one uninterrupted year. Dominant pancreatic strictures are defined by presence of at least one of the following characteristics: upstream MPD dilatation ≥6mm in diameter, prevention of contrast medium outflow alongside a 6-Fr catheter inserted upstream from the stricture, or abdominal pain during continuous infusion of a naso-pancreatic catheter inserted upstream from the stricture with 1L saline for 12–24hours. Pancreatic duct stents decompress the MPD and persistently dilate the stricture relieving pain and may improve the exocrine pancreatic function [14]. Numerous studies have demonstrated pain relief [28]. In a meta-analysis involving 1498 patients, 88% had immediate pain relief and 67% had long-term pain relief with endotherapy for pancreatic strictures with a 7.85% complication rate [29].

Multiple side-by-side stents and self-expandable metal stents (SEMSs) can be used for refractory strictures. Fully covered SEMSs have been demonstrated to offer better pain relief results over the uncovered and partially covered types, though further studies need to be conducted due to the associated potential complications [14]. Endoscopic ultrasonography can facilitate drainage of symptomatic MPD obstruction with failed trans-papillary approach with either the Rendezvous technique (puncturing the MPD through the gastric or duodenal wall and advancing a guidewire into the MPD to proceed with trans-papillary drainage) or through transmural drainage through a stent [14].

Malignancy should be ruled out before stent dilatation therapy.

9. Role of EUS and ERCP in the diagnosis of chronic pancreatitis

The diagnosis of chronic pancreatitis is based on altered pancreatic morphology and function. However, there is variation in the imaging findings using different modalities among patients with clinical features suggestive of chronic pancreatitis which sometimes delays diagnosis.

The American College of Gastroenterology (ACG) recommends cross-sectional imaging such as MRI or CT as first-line in the diagnosis of chronic pancreatitis in combination with careful history, physical examination, exposure risk, direct and/or indirect pancreatic function tests. These are preferred over ERCP and EUS due to the less invasiveness, objectivity, availability and cost differences. Endoscopic ultrasound can however be utilized if the findings from the cross-sectional imaging are in question. If EUS is inconclusive, secretin-enhanced magnetic resonance cholangiopancreatography (s-MRCP) or secretin- enhanced EUS are recommended [30]. A systematic review and meta-analysis on diagnostic performance of imaging modalities in chronic pancreatitis compared the sensitivity and specificity estimates of EUS, ERCP, MRI and CT, with no significant differences noted. Sensitivities for ERCP, EUS, MRI and CT reported were 82%; 95%CI: 76–87%), 81% (95%CI: 70–89%), 78% (95%CI: 69–85%), and 75% (95%CI: 66–83%), respectively and specificities, 94%; 95%CI: 87–98%), 90%; 95%CI: 82–95%), 96%; 95%CI: 90–98%) and 91%; 95% CI: 81–96%) respectively [31]. In the same study, abdominal ultrasonography was reported to have the lowest accuracy in diagnosing chronic pancreatitis. EUS can detect pancreatic parenchymal and ductal changes with high sensitivity and specificity producing high resolution ultrasonographic images due to the close proximity of the pancreas to the gastric and duodenal lumen.

A total of ten EUS criteria have been proposed by the International Working Group for Minimum Standard Terminology in Gastrointestinal Endoscopy for diagnosing chronic pancreatitis including five parenchymal criteria (hyperechoic foci, hyperechoic strands, parenchymal lobularity, cysts, calcifications) and five ductal criteria (pancreatic duct dilation, pancreatic duct irregularity, hyperechoic pancreatic duct walls, visible pancreatic side branches, intraductal calcifications) [32]. Diagnostic probability depends on the number of criteria observed, presence of two or less rules out chronic pancreatitis, presence of five or more criteria provides and definitive diagnosis, and presence of two to five criteria is indeterminate requiring pancreatic function tests. Some of the pancreatic changes seen during EUS have however been also associated with advanced age, smoking, obesity in the absence of chronic pancreatitis. EUS is operator dependant with poor inter-observer agreement which affects the reliability and standardization of EUS interpretation [33].

The Rosemont criteria was developed by a group of 32 experienced endosonographers in an attempt to harmonize and standardize the EUS based diagnosis of chronic pancreatitis. Ductal and parenchymal EUS findings are divided into major A, major

Parenchyma	Duct
Hyperechoic foci with acoustic shadows (major A); body/tail	Stones in the duct (major A)
Honeycomb-like lobulation (major B); body/tail	Irregular duct (minor); body/tail
Lobulation without honeycombing (minor); body/tail	Dilated side ducts (minor); body/tail
Hyperechoic foci without acoustic shadows (minor); body/tail	Dilated main duct (minor); body/tail
Cysts (minor)	Hyperechoic contours on the main duct (minor); body/tail
Echo-dense septa (minor); body/tail	

Table 1.
Rosemont criteria for endoscopic ultrasound diagnosis of chronic pancreatitis [34].

Assessment	Criteria
Consistent with CP	A. 1 major A + ≥ 3 minor B. 1 major A + 1 major B C. 2 major A
Suggestive of CP	A. 1 major A + < 3 minor B. 1 major B + ≥ 3 minor C. ≥ 5 minor
Indeterminate for CP	A. 3 to 4 minor, no major B. Major B +/− < 3 minor
Normal	A. <3 minor, no major

Table 2.
Interpretation of the Rosemont criteria [34].

B and minor criteria with different weight to different findings. Based on the number and character of positive EUS criteria, EUS evaluation is classified as "consistent with CP", "suggestive of CP", "indeterminate for CP", or "normal" [34]. However, the Rosemont criteria does not improve the inter-observer agreement compared to the standard EUS criteria [34] (**Tables 1** and **2**).

Diagnosis of early chronic pancreatitis presents a clinical challenge. EUS has been shown to detect some of the early features of chronic pancreatitis not detected by other imaging modalities [35]. ERCP remains a last-line diagnostic test and should be rarely used outside of therapeutic purposes.

Currently, histology is the gold standard for diagnosing early and late stages of chronic pancreatitis but not routinely done due to considerations of safety in obtaining samples from the pancreas. EUS is useful in obtaining pancreatic biopsies for histopathological diagnosis of chronic pancreatitis and other causative factors like pancreatic masses, autoimmune hepatitis. EUS-guided Fine Needle Aspiration (FNA) or Fine Needle Biospy (FNB) can be utilized to obtain biopsies for cytological and histological evaluation especially for cystic and mass lesions [36–39].

10. ERCP complications

ERCP alone or with the different therapeutic interventions is associated with different complications including pancreatitis, hemorrhage, infections, perforation and cardiopulmonary events. Other miscellaneous complications such as ileus, pneumothorax, pneumomediastinum, portal venous air, stent migration, liver abscess, biliary or pancreatic duct fistulae among others have also been reported but are very rare [40]. Their severity can range from mild to severe requiring hospitalization and possible permanent disability or death [41].

Three well studied interventions have demonstrated effectiveness in reduction of post-ERCP pancreatitis. These include:

10.1 Guidewire cannulation

Cannulation of the bile duct and pancreatic duct using a guidewire inserted through a catheter has been shown to significantly reduce the incidence of post-ERCP pancreatitis when compared with the conventional contrast cannulation [42–44]. Guidewire cannulation reduces post-ERCP pancreatitis by avoiding hydrostatic injury to the pancreas that may occur contrast injection and by reducing the need for precut sphincterotomy.

10.2 Pancreatic duct stents

In a meta-analysis evaluating 4 randomized prospective trials by Andriulli et al. [45] pancreatic duct stent placement had a twofold reduction in the incidence of post-ERCP pancreatitis (24.1% vs. 12%; P = 0.009; odds ratio: 0.44, 95% confidence interval: 0.24–0.81). Pancreatic duct stent insertion is technically difficult and there is need for follow-up evalutation to ensure passage or removal and associated with potential pancreatic ductal injuries. Insertion failure rates ranging from 4 to 10% have been reported and a higher incidence of severe pancreatitis among patients with failed pancreatic duct stenting [45–47].

10.3 Rectal non-steroidal anti-inflammatory drugs (NSAIDs)

Several drugs have been investigated for pharmaco-prophylaxis of post-ERCP pancreatitis. Of all drugs investigated, rectal NSAIDs have proved to be most effective at preventing post-ERCP pancreatitis [48–56].

11. Therapeutic role of ERCP and EUS in chronic pancreatitis

Chronic pancreatitis is a long standing painful inflammatory condition leading to progressive and irreversible pancreatic parenchymal damage and if not treated may result in either exocrine, endocrine insufficiency or both. This condition can be debilitating and severely affect the quality of life of these patients since most of them are either in and out of hospital, are on pain relieving medications, some may need enzyme supplementation and those that ultimately develop diabetes mellitus will have to be on oral hypoglycemic medications or insulin injections for life. Chronic pancreatitis may lead to stricture formation at the ampullary region leading to upstream dilatation of both the CBD and main pancreatic duct [57].

This ampullary strictures can also lead to both choledocholithiasis and main pancreatic duct stone formation further worsening the patient's symptoms. Other common complications of chronic pancreatitis include; pancreatic inflammatory space occupying lesions, pancreatic pseudocysts, walled of pancreatic necrosis can occur in either acute, subacute and rarely chronic pancreatitis. In cases where there is no known identifiable cause of chronic pancreatitis, empiric therapy is initiated targeting to pain, exocrine and endocrine pancreatic insufficiencies. Failure of empiric therapy will most likely lead to identifiable causes or complications of chronic pancreatitis like main pancreatic duct stones, dominant pancreatic duct stricture, pancreatic pseudocysts, walled of pancreatic necrosis and sometimes benign or malignant pancreatic neoplasms [58].

Pancreatic ductal stones can be spontaneously expelled. But when they persist ERCP + ES with or without stenting is done, the stones are extracted during ERCP and incase of failure of stone extraction by dormie baskets or stone extraction balloon catheters, mechanical or ESWL can be attempted. If the endotherapy options fail then open or laparoscopic surgical intervention is done.

Dominant pancreatic ductal strictures are managed based on the location and etiology, short strictures at the ampullar can be treated with either ERCP + ES with stenting or ampullectomy in case of small ampullary lesions causing ampullary strictures. Distal pancreatic ductal strictures will warrant endoscopically placing the stents across the stricture either via trans-papillary approach or a rendezvous approach. Failure in endotherapy will necessitate surgical intervention [59].

Pancreatic pseudocyst if asymptomatic and small are managed conservatively for at least 4 to 6 weeks. Large symptomatic pancreatic pseudocysts can be drained endoscopically during ERCP via the trans-papillary approach with stent insertion. They can also be drained via the trans-mural approach with the aid of endoscopic ultrasound guidance into the stomach, duodenum or proximal jejunum. EUS identifies the pseudocyst, maturity of the cyst wall, vascularity of the surrounding structures and helps in guided and safe creation of the cysto-gastrostomy or cysto-enterostomy with stent insertion. Endoscopic placement of the stent across the endoscopically created cysto-enterostomy ensures adequate pseudocysts drainage hence minimizing recurrence. Ultrasound guided percutaneous drainage can be done but increases the chances of a persistent pancreatico-cutaneous fistula formation. In case of failure of endoscopic drainage, open or laparoscopic surgical intervention can be done. Walled off pancreatic necrosis in the setting of chronic pancreatitis can be drained in the same way as pancreatic pseudocysts. The endoscope can be inserted into the cavity of the pancreatic necrosis cavity and the necrosectomy is done under direct vision after dilatation of the cysto-enterostomy. Stents are left across the cysto-enterostomy. Failure of endoscopic interventions may then warrant open or laparoscopic surgical intervention [60].

Endoscopic ultrasound in important in diagnosis of benign or malignant pancreatic neoplasms, sample can be taken for histological diagnosis and then a decision on the most appropriate management approach is chosen. Benign small asymptomatic pancreatic lesions less than 2 cm can be followed up with repeat EUS 3–6 months intervals. For symptomatic benign and malignant pancreatic lesions irrespective of the size will need endoscopic, laparoscopic or open resection with aim of obtaining clear resection margins post intervention. Small symptomatic lesions at the ampullar may undergo endoscopic ampullectomy but large lesions will necessitate surgical intervention [61].

12. Conclusion

ERCP and EUS are important in the management of both acute and chronic pancreatitis and its complications after failed empiric therapy. Endotherapy has the advantage of cosmesis, short hospital stay and decreased morbidity and mortality. Where endotherapy is unsuccessful or the cause of the pancreatitis is a large symptomatic malignant lesion, laparoscopic or surgical intervention will surfice.

Conflict of interest

None.

Author details

Michael Okello[1,2]* and Derick Kayondo[1]

1 Department of Surgery, Uganda Martyrs Hospital Lubaga, Kampala City, Uganda

2 Department of Anatomy, Makerere University College of Health Sciences, Kampala City, Uganda

*Address all correspondence to: dr.okelloaleleu@gmail.com

References

[1] McCune WS, Shorb PE, Moscovitz H. Endoscopic cannulation of the ampulla of vater: A preliminary report. Annals of Surgery. 1968;**167**(5):752-756

[2] Acosta JM, Ledesma CL. Gallstone migration as a cause of acute pancreatitis. The New England Journal of Medicine. 1974;**290**(9):484-487

[3] Tenner S, Baillie J, DeWitt J, Vege SS. American College of Gastroenterology guideline: Management of acute pancreatitis. The American Journal of Gastroenterology. 2013;**108**(9):1400-1415 1416

[4] Manes G, Paspatis G, Aabakken L, Anderloni A, Arvanitakis M, Ah-Soune P, et al. Endoscopic management of common bile duct stones: European Society of Gastrointestinal Endoscopy (ESGE) guideline. Endoscopy. May 2019;**51**(5):472-491. DOI: 10.1055/a-0862-0346. Epub 2019 Apr 3. PMID: 30943551

[5] van Geenen E-JM, van Santvoort HC, Besselink MGH, van der Peet DL, van Erpecum KJ, Fockens P, et al. Lack of consensus on the role of endoscopic retrograde cholangiography in acute biliary pancreatitis in published meta-analyses and guidelines: A systematic review. Pancreas. 2013;**42**(5):774-780

[6] Neoptolemos JP, Carr-Locke DL, London NJ, Bailey IA, James D, Fossard DP. Controlled trial of urgent endoscopic retrograde cholangiopancreatography and endoscopic sphincterotomy versus conservative treatment for acute pancreatitis due to gallstones. Lancet. 1988;**2**(8618):979-983

[7] Fan ST, Lai EC, Mok FP, Lo CM, Zheng SS, Wong J. Early treatment of acute biliary pancreatitis by endoscopic papillotomy. The New England Journal of Medicine. 1993;**328**(4):228-232

[8] Fölsch UR, Nitsche R, Lüdtke R, Hilgers RA, Creutzfeldt W. Early ERCP and papillotomy compared with conservative treatment for acute biliary pancreatitis. The German study group on acute biliary pancreatitis. The New England Journal of Medicine. 1997;**336**(4):237-242

[9] Heinrich S, Schäfer M, Rousson V, Clavien PA. Evidence-based treatment of acute pancreatitis: A look at established paradigms. Annals of Surgery. Feb 2006;**243**(2):154-168. DOI: 10.1097/01.sla.0000197334.58374.70. PMID: 16432347; PMCID: PMC1448904

[10] Moretti A, Papi C, Aratari A, Festa V, Tanga M, Koch M, et al. Is early endoscopic retrograde cholangiopancreatography useful in the management of acute biliary pancreatitis? A meta-analysis of randomized controlled trials. Digestive and Liver Disease. 2008;**40**(5):379-385

[11] Working Group IAP/APA Acute Pancreatitis Guidelines. IAP/APA evidence-based guidelines for the management of acute pancreatitis. Pancreatology. 2013;**13**(4 Suppl 2):e1-e15

[12] Cavdar F, Yildar M, Tellioğlu G, Kara M, Tilki M, Titiz Mİ. Controversial issues in biliary pancreatitis: When should we perform MRCP and ERCP? Pancreatology. 2014;**14**:411-414

[13] Acosta JM, Katkhouda N, Debian KA, Groshen SG, Tsao-Wei DD, Berne TV. Early ductal decompression versus conservative management for gallstone pancreatitis with ampullary obstruction: A prospective randomized clinical trial. Annals of Surgery. 2006;**243**(1):33-40

[14] Dumonceau J-M, Delhaye M, Tringali A, Arvanitakis M, Sanchez-Yague A, Vaysse T, et al. Endoscopic treatment of chronic pancreatitis: European Society of Gastrointestinal Endoscopy (ESGE) guideline - updated august 2018. Endoscopy. 2019;**51**(2):179-193

[15] Saritaş Ü, Üstündağ Y. Endoscopic retrograde Cholangiopancreatography in acute biliary pancreatitis. In: Yan Q, editor. Recent Advances in Pancreatitis. Rijeka: IntechOpen; 2021. DOI: 10.5772/intechopen.96545

[16] Lee SP, Nicholls JF, Park HZ. Biliary sludge as a cause of acute pancreatitis. The New England Journal of Medicine. 1992;**326**(9):589-593

[17] Saraswat VA, Sharma BC, Agarwal DK, Kumar R, Negi TS, Tandon RK. Biliary microlithiasis in patients with idiopathic acute pancreatitis and unexplained biliary pain: Response to therapy. Journal of Gastroenterology and Hepatology. 2004;**19**(10):1206-1211

[18] Elta G-H. Sphincter of Oddi dysfunction and bile duct microlithiasis in acute idiopathic pancreatitis. World Journal of Gastroenterology. 2008;**14**(7):1023-1026

[19] Canlas KR, Branch MS. Role of endoscopic retrograde cholangiopancreatography in acute pancreatitis. World Journal of Gastroenterology. 2007;**13**(47):6314-6320

[20] Wehrmann T. Long-term results (≥ 10 years) of endoscopic therapy for sphincter of Oddi dysfunction in patients with acute recurrent pancreatitis. Endoscopy. Mar 2011;**43**(3):202-207. DOI: 10.1055/s-0030-1255922. Epub 2010 Nov 24. PMID: 21108172

[21] Saad AM, Fogel EL, McHenry L, Watkins JL, Sherman S, Lazzell-Pannell L, et al. Pancreatic duct stent placement prevents post-ERCP pancreatitis in patients with suspected sphincter of Oddi dysfunction but normal manometry results. Gastrointestinal Endoscopy. 2008;**67**(2):255-261

[22] Khristenko E, Tjaden C, Klauß M. Pancreas divisum and pancreatitis. Der Radiologe. 2021;**61**(6):541-547

[23] Gutta A, Fogel E, Sherman S. Identification and management of pancreas divisum. Expert Review of Gastroenterology & Hepatology. 2019;**13**(11):1089-1105

[24] Larsen M, Kozarek R. Management of pancreatic ductal leaks and fistulae. Journal of Gastroenterology and Hepatology. 2014;**29**(7):1360-1370

[25] Singhal S, Rotman SR, Gaidhane M, Kahaleh M. Pancreatic fluid collection drainage by endoscopic ultrasound: An update. Clinical Endoscopy. 2013;**46**(5):506-514

[26] Hao W, Chen Y, Jiang Y, Yang A. Endoscopic versus laparoscopic treatment for pancreatic Pseudocysts: A systematic review and meta-analysis. Pancreas. 2021;**50**:788-795

[27] Sanders DJ, Bomman S, Krishnamoorthi R, Kozarek RA. Endoscopic retrograde cholangiopancreatography: Current practice and future research. World Journal of Gastrointestine Endoscopy. 2021;**13**(8):260-274

[28] Binmoeller KF, Jue P, Seifert H, Nam WC, Izbicki J, Soehendra N. Endoscopic pancreatic stent drainage in chronic pancreatitis and a dominant stricture: Long-term results. Endoscopy. 1995;**27**(9):638-644

[29] Jafri M, Sachdev A, Sadiq J, Lee D, Taur T, Goodman A, et al. Efficacy of

Endotherapy in the treatment of pain associated with chronic pancreatitis: A systematic review and meta-analysis. Journal of the Pancreas: JOP. 2017;**18**(2):125-132

[30] Gardner TB, Adler DG, Forsmark CE, Sauer BG, Taylor JR, Whitcomb DC. ACG Clinical Guideline: Chronic Pancreatitis. 2020;**115**:3

[31] Issa Y, Kempeneers MA, van Santvoort HC, Bollen TL, Bipat S, Boermeester MA. Diagnostic performance of imaging modalities in chronic pancreatitis: A systematic review and meta-analysis. European Radiology. 2017;**27**(9):3820-3844

[32] Iglesias-García J, Lariño-Noia J, Lindkvist B, Domínguez-Muñoz JE. Endoscopic ultrasound in the diagnosis of chronic pancreatitis. Rev Esp enfermedades Dig organo Of la Soc Esp Patol Dig. 2015;**107**(4):221-228

[33] Anaizi A, Hart PA, Conwell DL. Diagnosing chronic pancreatitis. Digestive Diseases and Sciences. 2017;**62**(7):1713-1720. DOI: 10.1007/s10620-017-4493-2

[34] Catalano MF, Sahai A, Levy M, Romagnuolo J, Wiersema M, Brugge W, et al. EUS-based criteria for the diagnosis of chronic pancreatitis: The Rosemont classification. Gastrointestinal Endoscopy. 2009;**69**(7):1251-1261

[35] Del Pozo D, Poves E, Tabernero S, Beceiro I, Moral I, Villafruela M, et al. Conventional versus Rosemont endoscopic ultrasound criteria for chronic pancreatitis: Interobserver agreement in same day back-to-back procedures. Pancreatology. 2012;**12**(3):284-287

[36] Cotton PB, Lehman G, Vennes J, Geenen JE, Russell RCG, Meyers WC, et al. Endoscopic sphincterotomy complications and their management: An attempt at consensus. Gastrointestinal Endoscopy. 1991;**37**(3):383-393. DOI: 10.1016/S0016-5107(91)70740-2

[37] Tryliskyy Y, Bryce GJ. Post-ERCP pancreatitis: Pathophysiology, early identification and risk stratification. Advances in Clinical and Experimental Medicine. 2018;**27**(1):149-154

[38] Badalov N, Tenner S, Baillie J. The prevention, recognition and treatment of post-ERCP pancreatitis. Journal of the Pancreas: JOP. 2009;**10**(2):88-97

[39] Freeman ML, DiSario JA, Nelson DB, Fennerty MB, Lee JG, Bjorkman DJ, et al. Risk factors for post-ERCP pancreatitis: A prospective, multicenter study. Gastrointestinal Endoscopy. 2001;**54**(4):425-434

[40] Chandrasekhara V, Khashab MA, Muthusamy VR, Acosta RD, Agrawal D, Bruining DH, et al. Adverse events associated with ERCP. Gastrointestinal Endoscopy. 2017;**85**(1):32-47

[41] Freeman ML. Pancreatic stents for prevention of post-endoscopic retrograde cholangiopancreatography pancreatitis. Clinical Gastroenterology and Hepatology. 2007;**5**(11):1354-1365

[42] Lella F, Bagnolo F, Colombo E, Bonassi U. A simple way of avoiding post-ERCP pancreatitis. Gastrointestinal Endoscopy. 2004;**59**(7):830-834

[43] Artifon ELA, Sakai P, Cunha JEM, Halwan B, Ishioka S, Kumar A. Guidewire cannulation reduces risk of post-ERCP pancreatitis and facilitates bile duct cannulation. The American Journal of Gastroenterology. 2007;**102**:10

[44] Cheung J, Tsoi KK, Quan W-L, Lau JYW, Sung JJY. Guidewire versus

conventional contrast cannulation of the common bile duct for the prevention of post-ERCP pancreatitis: A systematic review and meta-analysis. Gastrointestinal Endoscopy. 2009;**70**(6):1211-1219

[45] Andriulli A, Loperfido S, Napolitano G, Niro G, Valvano MR, Spirito F, et al. Incidence rates of post-ERCP complications: A systematic survey of prospective studies. The American Journal of Gastroenterology. 2007;**102**(8):1781-1788

[46] Rashdan A, Fogel EL, McHenry L Jr, Sherman S, Temkit M, Lehman GA. Improved stent characteristics for prophylaxis of post-ERCP pancreatitis. Clinical Gastroenterology and Hepatology. 2004;**2**(4):322-329

[47] Andriulli A, Forlano R, Napolitano G, Conoscitore P, Caruso N, Pilotto A, et al. Pancreatic duct stents in the prophylaxis of pancreatic damage after endoscopic retrograde cholangiopancreatography: A systematic analysis of benefits and associated risks. Digestion. 2007;**75**(2-3):156-163

[48] Elmunzer BJ, Waljee AK, Elta GH, Taylor JR, Fehmi SMA, Higgins PDR. A meta-analysis of rectal NSAIDs in the prevention of post-ERCP pancreatitis. Gut. 2008;**57**(9):1262-1267

[49] Murray B, Carter R, Imrie C, Evans S, O'Suilleabhain C. Diclofenac reduces the incidence of acute pancreatitis after endoscopic retrograde cholangiopancreatography. Gastroenterology. 2003;**124**(7):1786-1791

[50] Khoshbaten M, Khorram H, Madad L, Ehsani Ardakani MJ, Farzin H, Zali MR. Role of diclofenac in reducing post-endoscopic retrograde cholangiopancreatography pancreatitis. Journal of Gastroenterology and Hepatology. 2008;**23**(7pt2):e11-e16

[51] Dumonceau J-M, Kapral C, Aabakken L, Papanikolaou IS, Tringali A, Vanbiervliet G, et al. ERCP-related adverse events: European Society of Gastrointestinal Endoscopy (ESGE) guideline. Endoscopy. 2020;**52**(2):127-149

[52] Anderson MA, Fisher L, Jain R, Evans JA, Appalaneni V, Ben-Menachem T, et al. Complications of ERCP. Gastrointestinal Endoscopy. 2012;**75**(3):467-473

[53] Christensen M, Matzen P, Schulze S, Rosenberg J. Complications of ERCP: A prospective study. Gastrointestinal Endoscopy. 2004;**60**(5):721-731

[54] Glomsaker T, Hoff G, Kvaløy JT, Søreide K, Aabakken L, Søreide JA. Patterns and predictive factors of complications after endoscopic retrograde cholangiopancreatography. The British Journal of Surgery. 2013;**100**(3):373-380

[55] Wang P, Li Z-S, Liu F, Ren X, Lu N-H, Fan Z-N, et al. Risk factors for ERCP-related complications: A prospective multicenter study. The American Journal of Gastroenterology. 2009;**104**(1):31-40

[56] Chawla S, Willingham FF. Cardiopulmonary complications of endoscopic retrograde cholangiopancreatography. Techniques in Gastrointestinal Endoscopy. 2014;**16**(4):144-149

[57] Mayerle J, Talukdar R, Beyer G, Reddy DN. Interventional and Endoscopic Therapy of Chronic Pancreatitis. Pancreapedia: Exocrine Pancreas Knowledge Base; 2016. DOI: 10.3998/panc.2016.28

[58] D'Haese JG, Ceyhan GO, Demir IE, Tieftrunk E, Friess H. Treatment options in painful chronic pancreatitis: A systematic review. HPB. 2014;**16**(6):512-521. DOI: 10.1111/hpb.12173

[59] Issa Y, van Santvoort HC, van Goor H, Cahen DL, Bruno MJ, Boermeester MA. Surgical and endoscopic treatment of pain in chronic pancreatitis: A multidisciplinary update. Digestive Surgery. 2013;**30**(1):35-50. DOI: 10.1159/000350153

[60] Udd M, Kylänpää L, Kokkola A. The role of endoscopic and surgical treatment in chronic pancreatitis. Scandinavian Journal of Surgery. 2020;**109**(1):69-78. DOI: 10.1177/1457496920910009

[61] Christodoulou DK, Tsianos EV. Role of endoscopic retrograde cholangiopancreatography in pancreatic diseases. World Journal of Gastroenterology. 2010;**16**(38):4755-4761. DOI: 10.3748/wjg.v16.i38.4755

Chapter 6

Endoscopic Management of Chronic Pancreatitis

Arda Yavuz

Abstract

Chronic pancreatitis (CP) is a progressive inflammatory disease with several complications. Endoscopic methods make essential contributions to diagnosis and treatment. Endoscopic ultrasound is considered the most sensitive method for diagnosing early CP. Symptoms related to CP, failure of medical therapy, pancreatic changes in imaging (obstructive stones, strictures, and main pancreatic duct [MPD] dilatation), and complications (strictures, pseudocyst, and disruption of MPD) require interventional endoscopic methods. Pancreatic duct stenting could be beneficial when the patient has a dominant stricture in the pancreatic head or a refractory MPD stricture. Before stenting, underlying malignancy should be ruled out by brush cytology. In refractory cases, multiple plastic stents or fully covered self-expanding stents are necessary. Extracorporeal shock wave lithotripsy can also be performed with or without endoscopic retrograde cholangiography for stones in the pancreatic duct. In this case, the stone characteristics, stricture, and exocrine function determine the procedure. Endoscopic ultrasound-guided transmural or transpapillary drainage may be performed for pseudocyst-related CP, which has a success rate similar to surgery. Endosonography-guided celiac plexus block can also be used to treat CP.

Keywords: chronic pancreatitis, pancreatic ductal stones, stricture, pseudocyst, endoscopic ultrasound, celiac plexus block

1. Introduction

Chronic pancreatitis (CP) is a relapsing inflammatory disease characterized by pain, fibrotic strictures in the pancreatic and biliary ducts, calculi in the pancreatic duct, and an increased malignancy risk. Abdominal pain, weight loss, nausea, diarrhea, oily stools, and bloating are the main symptoms of this disease. Exocrine and endocrine insufficiency generally occurs during the late phases of the disease. The annual incidence rate is 5–12/100,000 people [1]. Alcohol consumption is the most common cause, accounting for approximately 65% of all cases [2]. Hereditary factors, congenital anatomical abnormalities, such as pancreas divisum or annulare, and autoimmune inflammation may play a role in the etiology.

Pain, which decreases the quality of life and causes high healthcare costs, is the main indication for endoscopic treatment when lifestyle changes and medical treatment fail. The first treatment step is the cessation of alcohol use and smoking for pain management, followed by the World Health Organization algorithm. Analgesics are the cornerstone at the beginning; however, when opioids are used, they may cause dependency, opioid-induced constipation, cognitive dysfunction, and opioid-induced hyperalgesia. In such cases, patients should be evaluated by a multidisciplinary team.

As interventional techniques are widely feasible and accepted, they play an important role in managing hepatobiliary diseases. Early diagnosis of CP is possible using endoscopic ultrasound (EUS)-based approaches, and interventional endoscopy can improve the complications of CP. In this chapter, we emphasize the use and importance of endoscopic modalities in the diagnosis and treatment of CP.

2. Endoscopic diagnosis of CP

CP is diagnosed when there is overt endocrine or exocrine dysfunction, atrophy, or calcification observed on imaging. However, these findings are observed in the later stages of the disease. EUS is highly beneficial for diagnosing early CP. Early diagnosis is essential for explaining symptoms, avoiding unnecessary explorations and therapies, investigating etiologies, adequate follow-up, explaining prognostic consequences, genetic evaluation, and appropriate therapy. Moreover, if there is a genetic mutation, total pancreatectomy and islet cell transplantation may be considered for malignancy risk.

EUS provides an opportunity to investigate the pancreatic parenchyma and ductal structures in detail. The parenchymal features of CP on EUS are hyperechoic foci, hyperechoic strands, lobularity, and cysts, and the ductal features are main ductal dilatation, duct irregularity, hyperechoic duct margins, visible side branches, and stones. In traditional EUS systems, the presence of five or more features reliably establishes the diagnosis of CP [3]. An international consensus panel, including 32 internationally recognized endosonographers, developed consensus criteria for EUS features of CP. In this Rosemont classification, the major criteria are hyperechoic foci with shadowing and main pancreatic duct (MPD) calculi and lobularity with honeycombing. Minor criteria are cysts, dilated ducts of ≥3.5 mm, irregular pancreatic duct contour, dilated side branches of ≥1 mm, hyperechoic duct wall, strands, non-shadowing hyperechoic foci, and lobularity with noncontiguous lobules **(Table 1)** [4].

	Parenchymal changes in CP	**Ductal changes in CP**
Major A	Hyperechoic foci with shadowing	MPD calculi
Major B	Lobularity with "honeycombing": ≥3 contiguous lobules measuring minimum 5 mm in length	
Minor	Lobularity without honeycombing	Irregular/ectatic MPD contour
	Hyperechoic foci without shadowing	≥3 dilated side branches
	Cysts	MPD dilatation > 3.5 mm body; >1.5 mm tail
	Hyperechoic stranding	Hyperechoic MPD margin

Consistent with CP: 1 major A and ≥3 minor features, 1 major A and 1 major B features, 2 major A features. Suggestive of CP: 1 major A and ≤3 minor features, 1 major B and ≥3 minor features. Indeterminate for CP: 3–4 minor, 1 major B alone or with <3 minor features. Normal: ≤2 minor without major features.

Table 1.
Rosemont classification.

Recent or active acute pancreatitis can cause overdiagnosis because of parenchymal hyperechoic strands and foci, lobularity, and hyperechoic duct walls. Acute inflammation of the pancreas can also obscure the underlying pancreatic mass. Therefore, EUS should be performed 4 weeks after an acute pancreatitis episode. Moreover, some of these EUS findings can be found normally in individuals as the age and among males, obese individuals, smokers, and alcohol consumers [5–8]. When the diagnosis of CP is debatable, EUS elastography, endoscopic pancreatic function test (ePFT), and distensibility of MPD can be combined with EUS to improve diagnostic success.

EUS elastography has been proposed as a novel and valuable modality for the evaluation of real-time tissue stiffness. It is mainly used in pancreatic tumors but is also highly beneficial in CP. Itoh et al. reported the correlation between parameters in EUS elastography (mean, standard deviation, skewness, and kurtosis) and histological fibrosis in the pancreas [9]. Iglesias-Garcia et al. showed the correlation between the strain ratio and Rosemont classification and exocrine dysfunction, evaluated by the carbon 13 mixed triglyceride breath test [10]. Homogenous stiffness on EUS elastography may also predict autoimmune pancreatitis. Both strain elastography and share wave elastography contributed to the diagnosis of CP using EUS.

The ePFT helped evaluate the exocrine function of the pancreas. In this procedure, gastroscopy was performed, and during the luminal examination, a test dose of secretin was intravenously administered. The gastric fluid was then aspirated as much as possible and discarded, and 3–5 cc post bulbar duodenal secretion was aspirated to rinse the gastric fluid from the suction channel. Furthermore, 3–5 cc duodenal fluid was aspirated as baseline collection; intravenous secretin (0.2 μg/kg) was administered slowly. Every 15 min, the duodenal aspirate was collected for 60 min. If the peak bicarbonate level was <80 mEq/L, then exocrine pancreatic insufficiency was considered. Its sensitivity was 92% and specificity 79% for early CP with normal imaging [11].

Inadequate distension of the MPD after secretin administration is another criterion used for the diagnosis of CP. Pancreatic duct dilatation after secretin stimulation lower than 50% of basal may be considered abnormal. In a study of 41 patients with clinically suspected CP, 77.3% had abnormal ductal compliance [12]. In current reports, additional criteria are suggested for EUS-based multimodal evaluation.

3. Pancreatic ductal stones

Unlike biliary stones, most pancreatic ductal stones are calcified and radiopaque. Stone prevalence increases during CP. In a multicenter study, 62% of 879 patients with CP reported calcified pancreatic stones. Heavy smokers (≥20 cigarettes/day), heavy drinkers (alcohol consumption of >80 g/day), and men have more pancreatic ductal stones than others [13].

Endoscopy, pancreatic sphincterotomy, and basket or balloon dilation allow stone extraction in only 9% of the patients. It is associated with stones of >10 mm, stone impaction, and a diffuse location [14]. Moreover, pancreatic mechanical lithotripsy has a threefold higher complication rate than biliary mechanical lithotripsy. These complications include trapped or broken baskets, traction wire fractures, and pancreatic ductal leak [15]. Furthermore, extracorporeal shock wave lithotripsy (ESWL) allowed successful pancreatic stone clearance in >80% of patients after failed stone extraction with endoscopy [16]. Therefore, primary endoscopy is reserved for selected patients with radiolucent stones or stones of <5 mm in size that are challenging to target with ESWL.

ESWL is a widely accepted treatment modality for radiopaque MPD stones when the MPD stone is larger than 5 mm and located in the head or body of the pancreas. Pancreatic stone clearance is achieved in 90% of the patients with CP; however, this can require multiple sessions [17]. Successful stone fragmentation was defined as stones broken into fragments of ≤2 mm, decreased stone density on radiography, increased stone surface, and heterogeneity of the stone. Ductal clearance could be complete, partial, or unsuccessful if the clearance of stones were <90%, 50–90%, or <50%, respectively. A meta-analysis reported that ESWL provided complete and partial clearance in 70% and 22% of patients, respectively, and pain was absent or mild for 2 years after ESWL in 52.7% and 33.4% of patients, respectively. After the procedure, the quality of life improved in 88.2% of patients [18]. If total stone clearance is achieved, pain relapse within the first 2 years after ESWL is rare. In the present case, half of the patients experienced stone recurrence. Small MPD stones (<5 mm) or radiolucent stones can be treated using endoscopic retrograde cholangiography (ERCP). The use of endoscopic therapy after ESWL is recommended when spontaneous clearance is not achieved. Additional endotherapy and ESWL had no benefit but were associated with longer hospital stays and higher treatment costs [19].

Large or multiple MPD stones or strictures are associated with the need for multiple ESWL sessions. In this case, pancreatic stenting before ESWL can decrease the need for additional ESWL procedures. Solitary stones, MPD stones in the pancreatic head, stones with a density on computed tomography (CT) scans of <820 HU, pancreatic stenting before the procedure, secretin administration before ESWL, and ERCP delayed by 2 days are related to better outcomes [20, 21]. Pancreatic pseudocysts are not related to MPD stone clearance [22]. The most common complication of ESWL is pancreatitis, asymptomatic hyperamylasemia, hematuria, mucosal injury, infection, skin erythema, tenderness, acute stone incarceration in the papilla, bleeding, and perforation could also be seen [23]. Contraindications for ESWL include non-correctable coagulopathy, pregnancy, and the presence of bone, calcified vessels, and lung tissue in the shockwave way [24].

Intracorporeal lithotripsy using electrohydraulic or laser lithotripsy under peroral pancreatoscopy, is recommended when ESWL is unavailable or stones are not fragmented after ESWL. A total of 43–100% of patients had successful MPD clearance in a systematic review. In the most extensive study of 38 patients (280 endoscopic therapy sessions, 88 of them with pancreatoscopy), complete and partial stone clearance was 24% and 10%, respectively [25, 26].

4. MPD strictures

In cases of stenosis in the MPD, possible malignancy should be ruled out using high-quality pancreatic CT or magnetic resonance cholangiopancreatography (MRCP). Brush cytology should be performed, and biopsy should be performed if necessary. A dominant MPD stricture is characterized by upstream MPD dilatation of ≥6 mm, prevention of contrast medium outflow alongside a 6-Fr catheter inserted upstream from the stricture, and abdominal pain during continuous infusion of a nasopancreatic catheter inserted upstream from the stricture with 1 L saline for 12–24 h. Technical success was defined as stent insertion across the dominant MPD stricture. This management aims to decompress the MPD, improves pain, dilates the stricture, and allows stone clearance after ESWL. A prospective non-randomized study on patients with dominant strictures reported less pain in the temporary pancreatic stenting group during a 5-year follow-up (15% vs. 50%) [27]. These strictures are generally single in >80% of the patients. Temporary single pancreatic stents provide 9–50% resolution and 67.5% pain relief [28, 29].

A refractory stricture was defined as symptomatic persistent dominant strictures or relapse after 1 year of single pancreatic stenting. Refractory strictures can be treated with multiple side-by-side stents, self-expanding metallic stents (SEMSs), or surgery. Temporary insertion of multiple side-by-side stents provided high stricture resolution and pain relief of 89.5% and 77.1%, respectively, during a 9.5-year follow-up [30]. SEMS insertion also achieved high pain improvement in 37–88% of all patients in a follow-up of 3–4 years [31]. Unlike SEMS, uncovered and partially covered stents are not suggested for migration risk.

Pancreatic sphincterotomy is mainly suggested if biliary drainage is necessary to facilitate MPD cannulation. Sphincterotomy is not mandatory for pancreatic stenting. Pancreatic stenting is performed mostly after ESWL if there is a pancreatic stone. The technical success of a single pancreatic stent is approximately 92%. In 18 series of 811 patients, the mean stenting duration was 10.6 months [32].

Multiple side-by-side pancreatic stents are another treatment option for refractory cases. Different stent designs are used: straight, winged, and s-shaped, with side holes. Stents with large side holes are suggested to have a low occlusion risk. The stent diameter is also critical. Patients with CP with ≤8.5-Fr pancreatic stents are 3.2 times more often hospitalized with abdominal pain than patients with CP with a 10-Fr pancreatic stent [33, 34].

The "on-demand" stent exchange strategy is based on clinical and laboratory evaluation at 6-month intervals, such as secretin-enhanced (S)-MRCP, abdominal ultrasound, abdominal radiography, and blood/urinary lipase analysis. However, this policy, in four series of 288 patients, reported a 5.2% rate of pancreatic sepsis [35]. Nevertheless, 12 series of 521 patients in whom the pancreatic stent was changed every 3 months regularly reported no septic complications [36].

Mild pancreatitis and worsening pancreatic pain are the most common short-term complications after plastic stenting, followed by sepsis, cholangitis, and post-sphincterotomy bleeding. During follow-up, proximal and distal stent migration was reported in 2.7% and 3.6% of the cases, respectively. Stent-induced ductal lesions were observed in 18% of the cases, and the mortality rate was 0.4% (7/1620). Complications after SEMS insertion include migration (15–46%), de novo strictures (16–27%), severe pain (7–20%), and stent removal (15%).

EUS-guided access and drainage is another treatment modality for patients with symptomatic MPD obstruction and failed transpapillary drainage. After puncturing the MPD through the gastric or duodenal wall, transpapillary drainage can be facilitated with a guidewire (rendezvous technique), transmural drainage with a plastic stent, or a fully covered SEMS (FCSEMS) can be used to achieve successful pain relief. This is one of the most challenging EUS-guided therapies. Failed EUS-guided access and drainage occur in 10% of cases, and complications such as severe pancreatitis, perforation, bleeding, and hematoma can occur [37]. This procedure is suggested only in tertiary centers after multidisciplinary discussion.

5. Benign biliary strictures

Biliary strictures occur during CP in 3–23% of all patients. Peribiliary fibrosis or pressure of the pancreatic pseudocyst (PPC) may play a role in pathophysiology. They can be asymptomatic or present with jaundice, cholangitis, or choledocholithiasis.

Jaundice could be resolved in 20–50% of patients in 1 month spontaneously [38]. However, secondary biliary cirrhosis is frequent (7.3%), and asymptomatic serum alkaline phosphatase and/or bilirubin for longer than 4 weeks predicts the need for endoscopic management [39]. As in all strictures of the hepatobiliary tract, malignancies should be excluded.

Single plastic stents are ineffective for the long-term management of biliary strictures. Multiple side-by-side plastic stents or FCSEMSs are widely used for endoscopic treatment. These stents have been suggested as the primary treatment for benign biliary strictures in the absence of associated lesions (such as inflammatory masses). Moreover, the success of the treatment was evaluated after 12 months or three endoscopic procedures. A single retrospective study comparing surgery and endoscopy reported that endoscopy had lower morbidity (21%, 83%) and success (15%, 66%) in the second year of treatment, which could be related to accepting incomplete resolution as a failure [40]. Uncovered SEMSs were not considered because of their poor long-term results. Multiple side-by-side plastic stents and FCSEMSs have similar success (88%, 90.9%) and morbidity (23.3%, 28.6%) rates [41]. If the stricture does not respond to endoscopic therapy, hepaticojejunostomy remains a valid treatment option.

6. Pancreatic pseudocysts (PPCs)

One-third of the patients with CP developed PPCs. In the evaluation, potentially malignant mucinous neoplasms should have been excluded. Transmural drainage, transpapillary drainage, or a combination of these techniques can be used in endoscopic treatment. The transpapillary route is only appropriate for half of the PPCs, which are small (<50 mm) and communicate with the MPD in the head or body of the pancreas [42]. Clinical success is defined as resolving the symptoms with complete resolution of PPC or a decrease in PPC to less than 2 cm [43]. Spontaneous regression of chronic PPCs is rare and typically occurs in PPCs of <4 cm. Symptomatic PPCs that cause abdominal pain, gastric outlet obstruction, early satiety, jaundice, weight loss, infection, or bleeding should be treated. Progressive growth of a PPC is an indication for some authors; however, others suggest follow-up for symptoms. If significant vessel compression occurs due to a PPC, the risk-benefit ratio should be checked before intervention.

Endoscopic drainage of PPCs has higher clinical success, shorter hospital stay than percutaneous drainage, and similar morbidity and recurrence rates [44]. Percutaneous drainage seems to be a better option when a PCC is not endoscopically accessible. A meta-analysis of 255 patients reported that surgery had a higher success rate, higher hospital cost, and extended hospital stay with similar morbidity and recurrence rates [45]. Current guidelines suggest endoscopic treatment for an uncomplicated PPC in CP over percutaneous or surgery, if accessible.

S-MRCP is a suggested method for evaluating the PPC and MPD anatomy before the procedure, which has an accuracy of >90% for diagnosing MPD rupture. In the management, transmural drainage is adequate in the absence of MPD rupture. In cases of partial rupture, treatment should include bridging the rupture with a stent. Complete MPD rupture (disconnected pancreatic duct syndrome) is associated with a high recurrence rate. Therefore, long-term indwelling of transmural double pigtail stents should be considered [46]. ERCP is regarded as the gold standard for diagnosing MPD rupture and carries an infection risk for a patient with a sterile PPC [47].

Transmural drainage can be performed using EUS or a conventional approach. EUS-guided transmural drainage has a higher technical success rate; however, there are no differences in the complications or clinical success. This difference occurs because of non-bulging collections, observed in approximately half of all PPCs [48]. Double pigtail plastic stents are generally preferred for PPCs. The number and diameter of these stents were not associated with clinical success [49]. biliary FCSEMSs could also be preferred when disconnected pancreatic duct syndrome is ruled out, and the duration is expected to be lesser than 6 weeks. A double pigtail plastic stent should be inserted through the biliary FCSEMS to prevent migration. Current guidelines suggest retrieval of transmural plastic stents at least 6 weeks after PPC regression; however, long-term indwelling of transmural plastic stents is needed for disconnected pancreatic duct syndrome. Retrospective studies have reported that long-term indwelling stents are highly effective and low PPC recurrence has been reported. PPC recurrence is associated with stent migration within 6 months and MPD disruption at the pancreatic head. Lumen-apposing metal stents can also be used for PPC in CP; however, it is less cost-effective than plastic stents.

Extrahepatic portal hypertension occurs during CP in ≥15% of all patients [50]. In this case, the EUS-guided transmural route was suggested. In two case series with 26 patients, the bleeding rate was 4% [51]. A pseudoaneurysm can occur in 1–10% of the cases during the course of CP [52]. Arterial embolization is suggested before the endoscopic drainage of a PPC.

7. Endosonography-guided celiac plexus block (CPB)

Once medical treatment options fail, persistent severe pancreatic pain can be treated endoscopically or surgically. The CPB can be used in patients with significant abdominal pain who have a poor general condition and have not responded to endoscopic treatment. In this technique, a combination of glucocorticoids and a long-acting local anesthetic (generally bupivacaine) can be administered using CT or EUS. EUS guidance is safer, more effective, and longer-lasting than CT. Bilateral injection (bupivacaine 0.25% [4 ml each side], followed by triamcinolone 80 mg [40 mg each]) and, central or unilateral injection (bupivacaine 0.25% [8 ml], followed by triamcinolone 80 mg) could be used. Bilateral injection seems to be an optimized distribution; however, supporting data are lacking.

It is unclear which patients derive the benefits of CPB. A long duration of pain may negatively affect the outcome because of permanent neuroplastic changes. Narcotic dependence is another factor that makes the treatment challenging. It is difficult to determine whether it is a hyperalgesia-related opioid or ineffective treatment, which also predicts a poor outcome. In a meta-analysis, it has been reported that EUS-guided CPB can relieve pain in 51–59% of patients [53]. However, it is reportedly inferior to surgical management. In a cohort study of 248 patients with CP, CPB was associated with pain relief in 177 patients (76%), with a median duration of 10 weeks [54]. The effect of CPB generally lasts for 3 months, after which the pain may worsen. It could be repeated for 3 or 6 months if it is beneficial in the initial celiac intervention. Nerve destruction may cause an increase in pain, hypotension, hemorrhage, infection, and neurological complications.

Celiac plexus neurolysis and absolute alcohol injection are used in pancreatic malignancies. However, it is not recommended for CP because of its potentially severe side effects. Due to the desmoplastic reaction, the possible future pancreatic surgery may get complicated. There is no routine recommendation or consensus for CPB or neurolysis for managing CP in the current guidelines.

8. Conclusions

The impact of endoscopy on managing CP is increasing. EUS-based criteria are the gold standard for diagnosing early CP. Early recognition of CP can change patients' futures. ESWL is the primary treatment of choice for patients with pancreatic stones. The strictures should be evaluated for possible malignancies. Plastic stents are feasible and cost-effective for treating benign strictures. Complications such as PPC can be successfully managed with transmural drainage. CPB is an alternative treatment option for opioid-resistant pancreatic pain. Surgery remains a treatment option after repeated procedures and in challenging refractory cases.

Conflict of interest

The author declares no conflict of interest.

Notes/thanks/other declarations

None.

Acronyms and abbreviations

CP	chronic pancreatitis
CPB	celiac plexus block
CT	computed tomography
ePFT	endoscopic pancreatic function test
ERCP	endoscopic retrograde cholangiopancreatography
ESWL	extracorporeal shock wave lithotripsy
EUS	endoscopic ultrasound
FCSEMS	fully covered self-expanding metal stent
MPD	main pancreatic duct
PPC	pancreatic pseudocysts
S-MRCP	secretin-enhanced magnetic resonance cholangiopancreatography

Appendices and nomenclature

None.

Author details

Arda Yavuz
Department of Gastroenterology, Istanbul Medeniyet University, Istanbul, Turkey

*Address all correspondence to: ardayavuz55@hotmail.com

References

[1] Yadav D, Lowenfels AB. The epidemiology of pancreatitis and pancreatic cancer. Gastroenterology. 2013;**144**(6):1252-1261

[2] Weiss FU, Laemmerhirt F, Lerch MM. Etiology and risk factors of acute and chronic pancreatitis. Visceral Medicine. 2019;**35**:73-81. DOI: 10.1159/000499138

[3] Conwell DL, Zuccaro G, Purich E, et al. Comparison of endoscopic ultrasound chronic pancreatitis criteria to the endoscopic secretin-stimulated pancreatic function test. Digestive Diseases and Sciences. 2007;**52**:1206-1210

[4] Catalano MF, Sahai A, Levy M. EUS-based criteria for the diagnosis of chronic pancreatitis: The Rosemont classification. Gastrointestinal Endoscopy. 2009;**69**(7):1251-1261. DOI: 10.1016/j.gie.2008.07.043

[5] Rajan E, Clain JE, Levy MJ, et al. Age-related changes in the pancreas identified by EUS: A prospective evaluation. Gastrointestinal Endoscopy. 2005;**61**:401-406

[6] Bhutani MS, Arantes VN, Verma D, et al. Histopathologic correlation of endoscopic ultrasound findings of chronic pancreatitis in human autopsies. Pancreas. 2009;**38**:820-824

[7] Al-Haddad M, Khashab M, Zyromski N, et al. Risk factors for hyperechogenic pancreas on endoscopic ultrasound: A case-control study. Pancreas. 2009;**38**:672-675

[8] Gardner TB, Levy MJ. EUS diagnosis of chronic pancreatitis. Gastrointestinal Endoscopy. 2010;**71**:1280-1289

[9] Itoh Y, Itah A, Kawashima H, et al. Quantitative analysis of diagnosing pancreatic fibrosis using EUS-elastography (comparison with surgical specimens). Journal of Gastroenterology. 2014;**49**:1183-1192

[10] Iglesias-Garcia J, Dominguez-Munoz JE, Castineira-Alvarino M, et al. Quantitative elastography associated with endoscopic ultrasound for the diagnosis of chronic pancreatitis. Endoscopy. 2013;**45**:781-788

[11] Ketwaroo G, Brown A, Young B, et al. Defining the accuracy of secretin pancreatic function testing in patients with suspected early chronic pancreatitis. The American Journal of Gastroenterology. 2013;**108**(8):1360-1366. DOI: 10.1038/ajg.2013.148

[12] Gardner TB, Purich ED, Gordon SR. Pancreatic duct compliance after secretin stimulation: A novel endoscopic ultrasound diagnostic tool for chronic pancreatitis. Pancreas. 2012;**41**:290-294

[13] Frulloni L, Gabbrielli A, Pezzilli R, et al. Chronic pancreatitis: Report from a multicenter Italian survey (PanCroInfAISP) on 893 patients. Digestive and Liver Disease. 2009;**41**:311-317

[14] Suzuki Y, Sugiyama M, Inui K, et al. Management for pancreatolithiasis: A Japanese multicenter study. Pancreas. 2013;**42**:584-588

[15] Thomas M, Howell DA, Carr-Locke D, et al. Mechanical lithotripsy of pancreatic and biliary stones: Complications and available treatment options collected from expert centers. The American Journal of Gastroenterology. 2007;**102**:1896-1902

[16] Farnbacher MJ, Schoen C, Rabenstein T, et al. Pancreatic duct

stones in chronic pancreatitis: Criteria for treatment intensity and success. Gastrointestinal Endoscopy. 2002;**56**:501-506

[17] Nguyen-Tang T, Dumonceau J-M. Endoscopic treatment in chronic pancreatitis, timing, duration and type of intervention. Best Practice & Research. Clinical Gastroenterology. 2010;**24**:281-298

[18] Moole H, Jaeger A, Bechtold ML, et al. Success of extracorporeal shockwave lithotripsy in chronic calcific pancreatitis management: A meta-analysis and systematic review. Pancreas. 2016;**45**:651-658

[19] Dumonceau J-M, Costamagna G, Tringali A, et al. Treatment for painful calcified chronic pancreatitis: Extracorporeal shock wave lithotripsy versus endoscopic treatment: A randomised controlled trial. Gut. 2007;**56**:545-552

[20] Ohyama H, Mikata R, Ishihara T, et al. Efficacy of stone density on noncontrast computed tomography in predicting the outcome of extracorporeal shock wave lithotripsy for patients with pancreatic stones. Pancreas. 2015;**44**:422-428

[21] Choi EK, McHenry L, Watkins JL, et al. Use of intravenous secretin during extracorporeal shock wave lithotripsy to facilitate endoscopic clearance of pancreatic duct stones. Pancreatology. 2012;**12**:272-275

[22] Li B-R, Liao Z, Du T-T, et al. Extracorporeal shock wave lithotripsy is a safe and effective treatment for pancreatic stones coexisting with pancreatic pseudocysts. Gastrointestinal Endoscopy. 2016;**84**:69-78

[23] Li B-R, Liao Z, Du T-T, et al. Risk factors for complications of pancreatic extracorporeal shock wave lithotripsy. Endoscopy. 2014;**46**:1092-1100

[24] Delhaye M. Extracorporeal shock wave lithotripsy for pancreatic stones. UpToDate. Accessed June 5. 2018

[25] Beyna T, Neuhaus H, Gerges C. Endoscopic treatment of pancreatic duct stones under direct vision: Revolution or resignation? Systematic review. Digestive Endoscopy. 2018;**30**:29-37

[26] Attwell AR, Brauer BC, Chen YK, et al. Endoscopic retrograde cholangiopancreatography with per oral pancreatoscopy for calcific chronic pancreatitis using endoscope and catheter-based pancreatoscopes: A 10-year single-center experience. Pancreas. 2014;**43**:268-274

[27] Seza K, Yamaguchi T, Ishihara T, et al. A long-term controlled trial of endoscopic pancreatic stenting for treatment of main pancreatic duct stricture in chronic pancreatitis. Hepato-Gastroenterology. 2011;**58**:2128-2131

[28] Topazian M, Aslanian H, Andersen D. Outcome following endoscopic stenting of pancreatic duct strictures in chronic pancreatitis. Journal of Clinical Gastroenterology. 2005;**39**:908-911

[29] Jafri M, Javed S, Sachdev A, et al. Efficacy of endotherapy in the treatment of pain associated with chronic pancreatitis: A systematic review and meta-analysis. Journal of the Pancreas. 2017;**18**:125-132

[30] Bove V, Tringali A, Valerii G, et al. Endoscopic dilation of pancreatic duct strictures in chronic pancreatitis with multiple plastic stents: Results in 48 patients. Gastrointestinal Endoscopy. 2017;**85**:AB236

[31] Tringali A, Vadalà di Prampero SF, Landi R, et al. Fully covered self-expandable metal stents to dilate persistent pancreatic strictures in chronic pancreatitis: Long-term follow-up from a prospective study. Gastrointestinal Endoscopy. 2018;**88**:939-946

[32] Weber A, Schneider J, Neu B, et al. Endoscopic stent therapy for patients with chronic pancreatitis: Results from a prospective follow-up study. Pancreas. 2007;**34**:287-294

[33] Buscaglia JM, DiMaio CJ, Pollack MJ, et al. Are large side holes associated with reduced rates of pancreatic stent occlusion? Results of a prospective study. Journal of the Pancreas: JOP. 2009;**10**:496-500

[34] Sauer BG, Gurka MJ, Ellen K, et al. Effect of pancreatic duct stent diameter on hospitalization in chronic pancreatitis: Does size matter? Pancreas. 2009;**38**:728-731

[35] Binmoeller KF, Jue P, Seifert H, et al. Endoscopic pancreatic stent drainage in chronic pancreatitis and a dominant stricture: Long-term results. Endoscopy. 1995;**27**:638-644

[36] Weber A, Schneider J, Neu B, et al. Endoscopic stent therapy in patients with chronic pancreatitis: A 5-year follow-up study. World Journal of Gastroenterology. 2013;**19**:715-720

[37] Chen Y-I, Levy MJ, Moreels TG, et al. An international multicenter study comparing EUS-guided pancreatic duct drainage with enteroscopy-assisted endoscopic retrograde pancreatography after Whipple surgery. Gastrointestinal Endoscopy. 2017;**85**:170-177

[38] Abdallah AA, Krige JEJ, Bornman PC. Biliary tract obstruction in chronic pancreatitis. HPB: The Official Journal of the International Hepato Pancreato Biliary Association. 2007;**9**:421-428

[39] Frey CF, Suzuki M, Isaji S. Treatment of chronic pancreatitis complicated by obstruction of the common bile duct or duodenum. World Journal of Surgery. 1990;**14**:59-69

[40] Regimbeau J-M, Fuks D, Bartoli E, et al. A comparative study of surgery and endoscopy for the treatment of bile duct stricture in patients with chronic pancreatitis. Surgical Endoscopy. 2012;**26**:2902-2908

[41] Haapamäki C, Kylänpää L, Udd M, et al. Randomized multicenter study of multiple plastic stents vs. covered self-expandable metallic stent in the treatment of biliary stricture in chronic pancreatitis. Endoscopy. 2015;**47**:605-610

[42] Barthet M, Lamblin G, Gasmi M, et al. Clinical usefulness of a treatment algorithm for pancreatic pseudocysts. Gastrointestinal Endoscopy. 2008;**67**:245-252

[43] Yoon SB, Lee IS, Choi MG. Metal versus plastic stents for drainage of pancreatic fluid collection: A meta-analysis. United European Gastroenterology Journal. 2018;**6**:729-738

[44] Khan M, Hammad T, Khan Z, et al. Endoscopic versus percutaneous management for symptomatic pancreatic fluid collections: A systematic review and meta-analysis. Endoscopy International Open. 2018;**6**:E474-E483

[45] Zhao X, Feng T, Ji W. Endoscopic versus surgical treatment for pancreatic pseudocyst. Digestive Endoscopy. 2016;**28**:83-91

[46] Kwon C-I, Gromski MA, Sherman S, et al. Clinical response

to dorsal duct drainage via the minor papilla in refractory obstructing chronic calcific pancreatitis. Endoscopy. 2017;**49**:371-377

[47] Costamagna G, Mutignani M, Ingrosso M, et al. Endoscopic treatment of postsurgical external pancreatic fistulas. Endoscopy. 2001;**33**:317-322

[48] Panamonta N, Ngamruengphong S, Kijsirichareanchai K, et al. Endoscopic ultrasound-guided versus conventional transmural techniques have comparable treatment outcomes in draining pancreatic pseudocysts. European Journal of Gastroenterology & Hepatology. 2012;**24**:1355-1362

[49] Lin H, Zhan X-B, Sun S-Y, et al. Stent selection for endoscopic ultrasound-guided drainage of pancreatic fluid collections: A multicenter study in China. Gastroenterology Research and Practice. 2014;**2014**:193562

[50] Bernades P, Baetz A, Lévy P, et al. Splenic and portal venous obstruction in chronic pancreatitis. A prospective longitudinal study of a medical-surgical series of 266 patients. Digestive Diseases and Sciences. 1992;**37**:340-346

[51] Rana SS, Sharma R, Ahmed SU, et al. Endoscopic ultrasound-guided transmural drainage of walled-off pancreatic necrosis in patients with portal hypertension and intra-abdominal collaterals. Indian Journal of Gastroenterology. 2017;**36**:400-404

[52] Evans RP, Mourad MM, Pall G, et al. Pancreatitis: Preventing catastrophic haemorrhage. World Journal of Gastroenterology. 2017;**23**:5460-5468

[53] Puli SR, Reddy JBK, Bechtold ML, et al. EUS-guided celiac plexus neurolysis for pain due to chronic pancreatitis or pancreatic cancer pain: A meta-analysis and systematic review. Digestive Diseases and Sciences;**54**:2330-2337

[54] Sey MS, Schmaltz L, Al-Haddad MA, et al. Effectiveness and safety of serial endoscopic ultrasound-guided celiac plexus block for chronic pancreatitis. Endoscopy International Open. 2015;**3**(1):E56-E59

Chapter 7

Pancreatic Pseudocyst

Christos Damaskos, Dionysios Prevezanos, Nikolaos Garmpis, Anna Garmpi, Gregory Kouraklis and Dimitrios Dimitroulis

Abstract

Pancreatic pseudocysts frequently occur in the context of acute or chronic pancreatitis and seldom appear as a post-surgical outcome or trauma. Complicated pancreatic pseudocysts represent extremely rare entities but still life-threatening situations, including infection, hemorrhage, rupture, pseudoaneurysms, pancreatic fistulas, obstructions, and splenic complications. Premature diagnosis, based on transabdominal ultrasonography or computed tomography, is crucial for the early therapeutic approach. Conservative treatment, surgical and endoscopic intervention consist the therapeutic options. Thus, management of the complicated pseudocysts demands a multidisciplinary team eligible to cope with complications that might even occur due to the intervention. Pancreatic pseudocysts represent a challenge for clinical doctors.

Keywords: pancreatic pseudocyst, differential diagnosis, complications, multidisciplinary approach, treatment

1. Introduction

Pseudocyst of the pancreas is a localized fluid collection that is rich in amylase and other pancreatic enzymes and is enclosed by a wall of non-epithelialized fibrous tissue. Pancreatic pseudocysts (PPCs) frequently occur in the context of acute or chronic pancreatitis and seldom appear as a postsurgical outcome or trauma. PPCs are less commonly related to acute pancreatitis compared to chronic pancreatitis, due to progressive ductal obstruction while the most common causative factor is alcohol consumption [1, 2]. Computed Tomography (CT) is the diagnostic modality of choice, as it considered to be superior to Ultrasound (US), providing more detailed information regarding the surrounding anatomy. It can demonstrate additional pathology, including pancreatic duct dilatation and calcifications, common bile duct dilatation, and extension of the pseudocyst outside the lesser sac. Complicated PPCs are extremely rare entities but still life-threatening situations, which affect the adjacent tissues of the pancreatic parenchyma. They can lead to infection, hemorrhage, rupture, pseudoaneurysms, pancreatic fistulas, obstructions, and splenic complications. Although they are well described, there is no consensus regarding the "gold-standard" therapy. Therapeutic approaches include conservative treatment(as a majority of cases have been resolved spontaneously), surgical and endoscopic intervention.

2. Historic review and classification for acute pancreatitis

Atlanta classification was the first classification for acute pancreatitis and was originally stated in 1992; giving the opportunity to the universal surgical community to have a common aspect regarding its definition [3]. However, soon this terminology proved to be inadequate and confusing and became outdated. In addition, definition of the pancreatic fluid collections was not well-established and there was huge variety among the surgeons [4]. Better comprehension of the etiology and the pathophysiology of the acute pancreatitis has led to revision of the Atlanta Classification for the acute pancreatitis, two decades later, correcting the aforementioned deficiencies. This revised classification differentiates the acute pancreatitis into two phases: early and late onset as well as the severity as mild, moderate, and severe [5].

Regarding the pancreatic and the peripancreatic fluid collections, terms such as "acute pseudocyst" and "abscess" were misleading and therefore discouraged. Instead, there was a clear distinction between collections that are consisted of sole fluid and those with debris (solid components due to necrosis). Another important factor affecting the categorization of the fluid collections is the presence of infection and certainly the duration of existence (**Figure 1**) [5]. In the Atlanta classification, PPC was described as a well-defined extra-pancreatic fluid collection with minimal solids, which lasts more than 4 weeks as the pancreatitis recedes.

3. Etiology

The appearance of PPC parallels that of pancreatitis and the etiology is strictly associated with the causes of pancreatitis. Typically, the PPCs form as a result of pancreatic duct disruption with subsequent fluid leakage or by the maturation of peripancreatic necrosis. Ninety percent of them occur in the context of pancreatitis, while only 10% are caused by trauma (surgery, gunshots, and blunt abdominal trauma) [6]. Regarding the acute pancreatitis, PPCs formation (approximately 15%) is infrequent

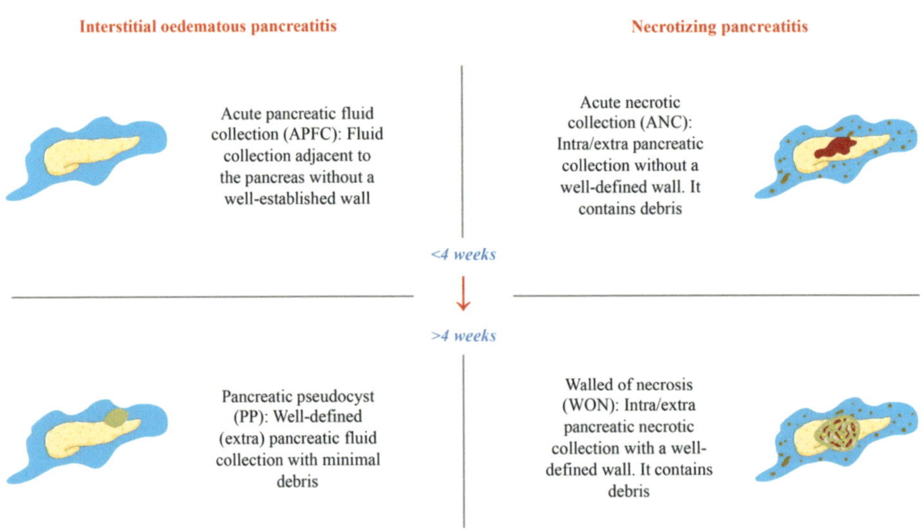

Figure 1.
Classification of pancreatic fluid collection.

in comparison with the chronic pancreatitis. Alcohol-associated pancreatitis appears to be the major causative factor in countries where alcohol consumption is high [7].

4. Pathogenesis

Several different procedures participate in the pathogenesis of the PPCs. In the cases that pseudocysts arise as a complication of severe acute pancreatitis, there is extravasation of pancreatic secretions due to disruption of the pancreatic duct. The gland necrosis leads to local fluid collection, which persists for more than 4 weeks as the inflammation recedes. Such pseudocysts usually contain enzymatic fluid and necrotic debris [8]. Concerning the pathogenesis of pseudocysts in chronic pancreatitis patients, at least two mechanisms may be involved. The cyst may develop as a consequence of progressive ductal obstruction by a protein plug, calculus, or localized fibrosis. In addition, a potentially acute exacerbation of the underlying disease can cause the cystic formation. Two-thirds of the patients with pseudocysts appear to have a connection between the pseudocyst and the pancreatic duct, while the rest do not have this exact finding and the cystic formation is caused due to the inflammatory reaction [9].

5. Classification system

Although PPC as a term is well-established, there is no classification system widely accepted. The first classification system was proposed by D'Egidio and Schein based on the underlying etiology of pancreatitis (acute or chronic), the pancreatic ductal anatomy and the presence of communication between the cyst and the pancreatic duct [10]. Using this classification system, the cyst may be divided into three distinct types:

- Type I, or acute "post-necrotic" pseudocysts, occur after an episode of acute pancreatitis and are associated with normal duct anatomy and rarely communicate with the pancreatic duct.

- Type II, also post-necrotic pseudocysts, occur after an episode of acute-on-chronic pancreatitis (the pancreatic duct is diseased, but not structured, and there is often a duct-pseudocyst communication).

- Type III, defined as "retention" pseudocysts, occur in chronic pancreatitis and are uniformly associated with duct stricture and pseudocyst-duct communication.

The latest classification system was proposed by Pan G. et al. based on the anatomical location and clinical manifestation of the pseudocysts, along with the relationship between the cyst and the pancreatic duct (**Table 1**) [11]. His aim was the selection of the optimal therapeutic approach for each stage.

6. Pancreatic pseudocysts differential diagnosis

Although PPCs are the most frequent cystic lesions, there are other malignant cystic lesions that can mimic the clinical manifestations of the PPCs. Malignant

Type	Description of pancreatic pseudocyst
I	<5 cm and without complications, symptom, and neoplasia
II	Suspected cystic neoplasia
III	The Location of pancreatic pseudocyst is uncinate
IIIa	Pseudocyst communication with the pancreatic duct
IIIb	Without communication between pseudocyst and pancreatic duct
IV	Location of pancreatic pseudocyst is head, neck and body
IVa	Exist communication between pseudocyst and pancreatic duct
IVb	Distance from the cyst to the gastrointestinal wall is <1 cm
IVc	Neither IVa nor IVb
V	Location of pancreatic pseudocyst is tail
Va	Splenic vein involvement or upper gastrointestinal bleeding
Vb	Distance from the cyst to the gastrointestinal wall is <1 cm, without splenic vein involvement or upper gastrointestinal bleeding

Table 1.
Pan G. et al. classification of pancreatic pseudocysts.

cystic lesions account for 10–15% of the pancreatic cysts [12]. It is well established, that imaging modalities alone can be misleading in diagnosing cystic malignancies due to the imaging similarities [13]. In general terms, the risk of potential malignancy in incidentally detected cysts is low [14]. The most common cystic malignancy is Branch Duct Intraductal Papillary Mucinous Neoplasm (BD-IPMN) [15]. Predictive factors for malignancy are the size of the cyst (>3 cm), dilated pancreatic duct, and the solid component associated with the cyst. Multiple cysts and cyst enlargement over time are not correlated with the appearance of neoplasm [14].

The distinction is important in order to provide the optimal therapy for the patient. The differential diagnosis should include serous cystic tumors, mucinous cystic neoplasms, solid pseudopapillary neoplasms, and the recently known Intraductal papillary mucosa neoplasm (IPMNs). In the context of absence of history of pancreatitis, the physicians should suspect malignancy and further diagnostic modalities such as image-guided aspiration/biopsy should be performed. Magnetic resonance cholangiopancreatography (MRCP) can visualize possible communication between the main pancreatic duct and a cystic lesion noninvasively. In addition, endoscopic ultrasound can provide further structure information in greater detail and facilitate aspiration or biopsy of smaller lesions [16].

7. Clinical manifestations

Patients with acute pancreatitis who are not treated within seven days or those whose symptoms reappear after a transient improvement period should be suspected of pancreatic pseudocysts. The clinical manifestations are strictly associated with the local mass effect. The symptoms and the signs are summarized in **Table 2**.

Frequency	Sign and symptom
Most frequent	Abdominal pain and early satiety
Uncomon	Fever, palpable mass, weight loss/anorexia (due to gastric duodenal compression), feeding intolerance
Rare	Jaundice (due to bile duct compression)

Table 2.
Signs and symptoms of pancreatic pseudocysts.

8. Radiological examinations

The golden standard radiological measure of the PPCs is the CT. It can visualize the size of the cyst, its shape as well as any possible association with the adjacent tissues. Also, bearing in mind that PPCs are a progressive disease, CT can facilitate the follow-up.

Regarding the US, it is a side-bed, inexpensive, and noninvasive radiological modality. Also, with its ability to measure blood flow, it is suitable to differentiate pseudoaneurysms or ruptures inside the PPC. Finally, US can serve as an imaging guide for further diagnostic and interventional methods. Despite these advantages, the most crucial problem is the visibility and the exposure of the pancreas and the peri-pancreatic region due to the bowel gas and the patient's weight. In addition, it is operator-dependent with a sensitivity in pancreatic fluid collections of approximately 75–93% [17].

Last but not least, magnetic resonance imaging (MRI) can also provide similar data for the PPCs. Its main advantage is the capacity for easier differentiation of the solid debris [18]. MRI also proved to be superior to CT in the prediction of a potential drainable peri-pancreatic fluid collection [19]. However, MRI is far more expensive than CT and its availability is limited at several institutions.

9. Pancreatic pseudocysts complications

Generally, peri-pancreatic fluid collections are sterile and most of the cases are resolved without any invasive intervention. Potentially, untreated pancreatic pseudocysts can cause life threatening complications including Infection, rupture, pancreatic fistulas and ascites, vascular complications (Pseudoaneurysm formation, Hemosuccus Pancreaticus, Splenic or Portal vein thrombosis), and splenic complications and local mass effect (Gastrointestinal, Urinary obstruction or biliary complications).

9.1 Infection

As aforementioned, peri-pancreatic fluid collections are sterile. Infected pancreatic pseudocysts occur in up to 10% of cases, usually spontaneously or after iatrogenic intervention (diagnostic or therapeutic manipulation) [20]. The most common species of pathogens that are frequently found in PPCs originated from the enteric flora and include E. coli, Klebsiella pneumoniae, Enterococcus spp., and, Enterobacter spp., less frequent are Pseudomonas aeruginosa, Streptococcus spp., Staphylococcus spp., and Bacteroides [21]. The route of the bacteria leading to infection in pancreatic pseudocyst is still unclear. Several mechanisms have been proposed, such as infection from the biliary tree or duodenum, translocation of bacteria from the gut, and hematogenous or lymphatic spread from other sites.

Since clinical manifestations may vary, infection should be suspected in any. patient with fever or suggestive signs or symptoms of sepsis. An infected pancreatic pseudocyst is accompanied by fever, shivering, and elevated white blood cell count. The presence of bubble gas sign on CT is a crucial finding for infection and the physician should be suspected. Nevertheless, US-guided aspiration (EUS-FNA) and sending the fluid for gram stains and cultures will provide the definitive diagnosis.

In addition, the results would provide information for the appropriate antibiotic treatment. If the acute infection is confirmed, then drainage should be performed by endoscopic, percutaneous, or surgical procedures.

9.2 Rupture

Rupture of the pancreatic pseudocyst can lead to a favorable outcome or a potentially life-threatening situation. Rupture to the adjacent gastrointestinal tract will lead to vomiting, diarrhea, melena, hematemesis, or hematochezia. However, rupture into the peritoneal cavity can cause severe peritonitis or hemorrhagic shock and pancreatic ascites. Its clinical manifestation includes severe abdominal pain, fever, food intolerance, tachycardia, and hypotension. Intraperitoneal hemorrhage from ruptured pancreatic pseudocyst is associated with an extremely high mortality rate (35.3%) [22]. The exact mechanism of rupture remains unknown. Possibly, erosion or disruption due to either severe inflammation or the activated lytic enzymes in the pseudocyst, in a superficial vessel may have weakened the pseudocyst wall, subsequently resulting in the spontaneous rupture of the pseudocyst [23]. The content of the pseudocyst (amylase, lipase, and other proteolytic enzymes) can cause erosion of the nearby viscera, thrombosis of the adjacent vessels, or further complications [24].

Traditionally, the optimal therapeutic choice is the internal drainage either through cysteogastrostomy or Roux-en-Y cysteojejunostomy [25]. Extensive local inflammation or incapability of identifying the cyst walls can lead to the failure of creation of the anastomosis. In these cases, external drainage and lavage of the peritoneal cavity can be achieved with safety [9]. Recently, another option, which was reported, is the endoscopic ultrasound-guided drainage and endoscopic ultrasound-guided gastrocystostomy with a fully covered self-expandable metallic stent [26]. However, the authors highlighted that can be useful in local fluid collection due to the ruptured pseudocyst.

Regarding the ruptured pseudocysts in nearby viscera, the literature recommends conservative treatment unless there is active bleeding, or the patient is febrile. The most common site seems to be the stomach, but there is not enough data to support this. Beside the conservative treatment, the authors recommend endoscopic intervention (potential clipping of bleeding vessels, stenting) as first choice of treatment and surgical intervention when endoscopic management is impossible (gastrectomy) [23, 27–29].

9.3 Pancreatic fistula and ascites

A big majority of patients with acute pancreatitis will develop pseudocysts, while only a small percentage of them will develop fistula or ascites as pseudocyst complications. There is no data regarding the mechanism for the creation of the fistula.

Fistulas are divided into two categories: internal which include fistulas associated with the adjacent viscera to the pseudocyst; andnd external, mainly due to iatrogenic manipulations. Connection from the pseudocyst to the stomach, colon, small intestine, bronchi, biliary tract, and esophagus have been described. Early recognition of this rare entity is crucial. CT, MRI, and MRCP have a principal role. In addition, fistulography has been proven trustworthy for a definitive diagnosis [30]. Like the aforementioned complications, a stepwise approach is the key starting from conservative treatment to endoscopic or surgical interventions.

The external pancreatic pseudocyst fistulas can mostly occur as a complication of the percutaneous drainage. On suspicion, any aspired fluid must be checked for amylase levels ensuring the diagnosis. Also, another option is to inject a contrast media through the drain or fistula to assess for a pancreatogram, which confirms the diagnosis. Initial treatment is considered to be conservative as in the majority of the cases, fistulas are resolved without any intervention [31]. Although external fistulas are iatrogenic complications, there are a few cases that have been reported with spontaneous pancreatocutaneous fistula [32, 33]. In both cases, pseudocyst occurred retroperitoneally with swelling at the left lumbar and left flank region accordingly. In the first case, conservative treatment was chosen while the second one underwent surgical drainage. Both cases had favorable outcomes.

Ascites are another complication of the pancreatic pseudocyst. In most of the cases (about 80%), ascites appears due to leakage of the pseudocyst in patients with chronic pancreatitis [34, 35]. Patients with pancreatic ascites usually refer to mild abdominal pain, decreased appetite, sense of satiety, and weight loss. One very important leading point is the medical history of patient, which must include chronic pancreatitis or a recent episode of acute pancreatitis. The diagnosis is set by drainage and the ascitic fluid has high amylase concentration (over 1000 IU/L) and protein concentration over 3 g/dl, which differentiates it from cirrhosis, tuberculosis, or malignancy [36]. Imaging modalities that could lead to diagnosis is the endoscopic retrograde cholangiopancreatography (ERCP) which is the “gold standard” to confirm the site of leakage; while in cases where ERCP is contraindicated, MRCP can define the anatomy of pancreatic duct and its abnormalities [37, 38]. Treatment of this entity concerns mainly the therapy of the pancreatic pseudocyst. Conservative treatment, drainage either internal (cystogastrostomy, cystojejunostomy, or cystoduodenostomy) or external and distal pancreatectomy when the leak is in the pancreatic tail are possible options [37].

9.4 Vascular complications

Patients suffering from pancreatic pseudocysts can potentially develop vascular complications, such as pseudoaneurysm formation within the cyst, splenic and portal vein complications.

Formation of pseudoaneurysm inside the pancreatic pseudocyst is a rare pathology and life-threatening situation with high mortality rates. The exact mechanisms are still under investigation, but three possible mechanisms have been proposed. Firstly, inflammation in conjunction with pancreatic enzymes could lead to erosion of pancreatic or peripancreatic artery and consequently the formation of pseudoaneurysm; communication of a pancreatic pseudocyst with a vessel; and lastly a pseudocyst eroding the bowel wall with bleeding [39, 40]. The symptoms are nonspecific, and even on suspicion the patient must undergo a thorough examination to avoid any rupture resulting in severe bleeding. Contrast-enhanced CT or angiography if the patient is stable is used for recognition of the vessel. In addition, angiography can be used for immediate angio-embolization after tracking the bleeding site. Endovascular interventions should be the first-line treatment [41]. In case of unsuccessful endovascular intervention, a surgical treatment should be performed. The general idea is drainage of the pancreatic pseudocyst and arterial ligation of the vessel that causes the pseudoaneurysm. Splenic artery is the most frequent vessel involved [42].

A pseudocyst can also be the cause of portal vein or splenic vein thrombosis. Pathophysiologically, local inflammation and complement system activation can contribute to thrombosis. In addition, pseudocyst can compress the portal or splenic vein leading to obstruction and consequently to portal hypertension. Treatment includes management of the pancreatic pseudocyst and its cause, e.g. lithrotripsy if choledocholithiasis exist, and management of the thrombosis. Anti-coagulation therapy, thrombolytic agents (urokinase), endovascular intervention (transjugular intrahepatic portosystemic shunt) as well as surgery have been described [43–45].

Last but not least, communication between the pseudoaneurysm and the pancreatic duct can result in severe bleeding to gastrointestinal tract through the ampulla of Vater. This life-threatening situation is called hemosuccus pancreaticus also known as wirsungorrhagia and pseudohemobilia. The most frequent clinical manifestation includes melena, hematochezia or hematemesis, symptomatic anemia, abdominal pain, nausea, and vomiting [46]. The "gold standard" diagnostic as well as therapeutic modality is the angiography identifying the causative vessel and applying the proper interventional method (stent placement and metallic coil embolization). In patients whose endoscopic intervention failed, or in those that are unstable, surgery is still an option without experiencing unwanted complications [47].

9.5 Splenic complications

Splenic rupture in acute and chronic pancreatitis accounts for 9% of the atraumatic splenic ruptures [48]. Especially, if a pancreatic pseudocyst occurs at the tail of the pancreas, the pancreatic enzymes and the inflammation can erode the splenic parenchyma secondary to hematoma. The main etiological factor is excessive alcohol consumption, while the majority of patients are referring to abdominal pain, nausea, vomiting, and lumbar pain [49]. Early recognition of this complication with CT and/or angiography is important for the immediate therapeutic approach, which is consisted of conservative management, percutaneous drainage, splenic artery embolization (hematoma exists without rupture), and splenectomy (when a rupture occurs) [50–52].

Other splenic complications, such as splenic artery pseudoaneurysm and splenic vein thrombosis are described in the "vascular complications" session.

9.6 Local mass effect

There have been reported cases in which the pancreatic pseudocyst caused compression to the adjacent viscera due to its huge size. Additionally, a big pancreatic pseudocyst can increase the intra-abdominal pressure leading to orthopnea, dyspnea, abdominal pain, and distention. Depending on the region of the cyst, the common bile duct and the poral vein or the splenic vein could be obstructed resulting in obstructive jaundice and portal hypertension (see session "vascular complications") accordingly [53, 54]. Endoscopic approach reducing the size of the cyst combined with stenting is the ideal treatment for this situation.

10. Conclusions

PPC is a frequent complication of acute or chronic pancreatitis. Maturation of the pseudocyst needs at least 2–6 weeks. In this short period of time, the majority of them are resolved without any invasive treatment. Patients with persistent symptoms should be examined thoroughly. Early recognition of the complication of the pancreatic pseudocyst is mandatory. An abdominal CT scan is the initial radiological modality. Multidisciplinary and stepwise approaches to evaluating the data properly will lead to favorable outcomes for the patient. The physicians should be suspicious of these aforementioned rare complications, which can potentially be fatal.

Author details

Christos Damaskos[1,2]*, Dionysios Prevezanos[1], Nikolaos Garmpis[2,3], Anna Garmpi[4], Gregory Kouraklis[5] and Dimitrios Dimitroulis[3]

1 Renal Transplantation Unit, Laiko General Hospital, Athens, Greece

2 N.S. Christeas Laboratory of Experimental Surgery and Surgical Research, Medical School, National and Kapodistrian University of Athens, Athens, Greece

3 Second Department of Propedeutic Surgery, Laiko General Hospital, Medical School, National and Kapodistrian University of Athens, Athens, Greece

4 First Department of Propedeutic Internal Medicine, Laiko General Hospital, Medical School, National and Kapodistrian University of Athens, Athens, Greece

5 Medical School, National and Kapodistrian University of Athens, Athens, Greece

*Address all correspondence to: damaskos@yahoo.gr

References

[1] Agalianos C, Passas I, Sideris I, Davides D, Dervenis C. Review of management options for pancreatic pseudocysts. Translational Gastroenterology and Hepatology. 2018;**3**:18

[2] Lerch MM, Stier A, Wahnschaffe U, Mayerle J. Pancreatic pseudocysts: Observation, endoscopic drainage, or resection? Deutsches Ärzteblatt International. 2009;**106**(38):614-621

[3] Bradley EL. A clinically based classification system for acute pancreatitis. Summary of the International Symposium on Acute Pancreatitis, Atlanta, Ga, September 11 through 13, 1992. Archives of Surgery. 1993;**128**(5):586-590

[4] Bollen TL, van Santvoort HC, Besselink MG, van Leeuwen MS, Horvath KD, Freeny PC, et al. The Atlanta classification of acute pancreatitis revisited. The British Journal of Surgery. 2008;**95**(1):6-21

[5] Banks PA, Bollen TL, Dervenis C, Gooszen HG, Johnson CD, Sarr MG, et al. Classification of acute pancreatitis--2012: Revision of the Atlanta classification and definitions by international consensus. Gut. 2013;**62**(1):102-111

[6] Muniraj T, Gajendran M, Thiruvengadam S, Raghuram K, Rao S, Devaraj P. Acute pancreatitis. Disease-a-Month. 2012;**58**(3):98-144

[7] Walt AJ, Bouwman DL, Weaver DW, Sachs RJ. The impact of technology on the management of pancreatic pseudocyst. Fifth annual Samuel Jason Mixter Lecture. Archives of Surgery. 1990;**125**(6):759-763

[8] Pitchumoni CS, Agarwal N. Pancreatic pseudocysts: When and how should drainage be performed? Gastroenterology Clinics of North America. 1999;**28**(3):615-639

[9] Habashi S, Draganov PV. Pancreatic pseudocyst. World Journal of Gastroenterology. 2009;**15**(1):38-47

[10] D'Egidio A, Schein M. Pancreatic pseudocysts: A proposed classification and its management implications. The British Journal of Surgery. 1991;**78**(8):981-984

[11] Pan G, Wan MH, Xie KL, Li W, Hu WM, Liu XB, et al. Classification and management of pancreatic pseudocysts. Medicine (Baltimore). 2015;**94**(24):e960

[12] Friedman AC, Lichtenstein JE, Dachman AH. Cystic neoplasms of the pancreas. Radiological-pathological correlation. Radiology. 1983;**149**(1):45-50

[13] Curry CA, Eng J, Horton KM, Urban B, Siegelman S, Kuszyk BS, et al. CT of primary cystic pancreatic neoplasms: Can CT be used for patient triage and treatment? AJR. American Journal of Roentgenology. 2000;**175**(1):99-103

[14] Scheiman JM, Hwang JH, Moayyedi P. American gastroenterological association technical review on the diagnosis and management of asymptomatic neoplastic pancreatic cysts. Gastroenterology. 2015;**148**(4):824-848

[15] Tanaka M, Fernández-del Castillo C, Adsay V, Chari S, Falconi M, Jang JY, et al. International association of pancreatology: International consensus guidelines 2012 for the management

of IPMN and MCN of the pancreas. Pancreatology. 2012;**12**(3):183-197

[16] Bounds BC, Brugge WR. EUS diagnosis of cystic lesions of the pancreas. International Journal of Gastrointestinal Cancer. 2001;**30**(1-2):27-31

[17] Dhaka N, Samanta J, Kochhar S, Kalra N, Appasani S, Manrai M, et al. Pancreatic fluid collections: What is the ideal imaging technique? World Journal of Gastroenterology. 2015;**21**(48):13403-13410

[18] Macari M, Finn ME, Bennett GL, Cho KC, Newman E, Hajdu CH, et al. Differentiating pancreatic cystic neoplasms from pancreatic pseudocysts at MR imaging: Value of perceived internal debris. Radiology. 2009;**251**(1):77-84

[19] Morgan DE, Baron TH, Smith JK, Robbin ML, Kenney PJ. Pancreatic fluid collections prior to intervention: Evaluation with MR imaging compared with CT and US. Radiology. 1997;**203**(3):773-778

[20] Byrne MF, Baillie J. Pancreatic fluid collections and pseudocysts in patients with acute pancreatitis. In: Forsmark CE, editor. Pancreatitis and Its Complications. Clinical Gastroenterology. Totowa, NJ: Humana Press Inc.; 2005

[21] Sabater-Orti L, Calvete-Chornet J, Lledó-Matoses S. Therapeutic approach to pancreatic abscess. Clinical Gastroenterology. 2007:149-155

[22] Sugimoto S, Murakami M, Ota T, Ichihara S, Naito M, Shimizu N. A case of intraperitoneal hemorrhage from ruptured pancreatic pseudocyst. Journal of Japan Surgical Association. 2005;**66**:3053-3057

[23] Urakami A, Tsunoda T, Kubozoe T, Takeo T, Yamashita K, Imai H. Rupture of a bleeding pancreatic pseudocyst into the stomach. Journal of Hepato-Biliary-Pancreatic Surgery. 2002;**9**(3):383-385

[24] Patidar Y, Sureka B, Singh VP, Bansal K, Maiwall R. Spontaneous rupture of intrahepatic pseudocyst into the inferior vena cava. Gastroenterology Report (Oxford). 2018;**6**(3):225-227

[25] Mujer MT, Rai MP, Atti V, Shrotriya S. Spontaneous rupture of a pancreatic pseudocyst. BML Case Reports. 2018;**2018**:bcr2018226296

[26] Park C, Kim TH, Chon HK. Successful endoscopic ultrasound-guided treatment of a spontaneous rupture of a hemorrhagic pancreatic pseudocyst. Clinical Endoscopy. 2021;**54**(5):763-766

[27] Madhyastha SP, Banda GR, Acharya RV, Balaraju G. Spontaneous rupture of pancreatic pseudocyst into the stomach. BML Case Reports. 2021;**14**(7):e244839

[28] Kanaan Z, Zhang A, Lilley K, Mutchnick M. Uncomplicated spontaneous rupture of a pancreatic pseudocyst into the stomach through a fistula: A case report and review of the literature. Pancreas. 2018;**47**(4):e22-e24

[29] Angelis A, Kykalos S, Garoufalia Z, Karatza E, Garmpis N, Damaskos C, et al. Management of a complicated pancreatic pseudocyst: Report of a case and review of the literature. Journal of the Pancreas. 2018;**19**(3):157-163

[30] Faccioli N et al. Role of fistulography in evaluating pancreatic fistula after pancreaticoduodenectomy. The British Journal of Radiology. 2012;**85**(1011):219-224

[31] Sikora SS, Khare R, Srikanth G, Kumar A, Saxena R, Kapoor VK. External pancreatic fistula as a sequel to management of acute severe necrotizing pancreatitis. Digestive Surgery. 2005;**22**(6):446-451

[32] Radojkovic M, Kovacevic P, Radojkovic D. Pancreatic pseudocyst with spontaneous cutaneous fistulization: Case report. Medicine (Baltimore). 2018;**97**(35):e12051

[33] Fitchett JM, Beaumont A, Davies IL, Lewis MH. An extreme presentation of pancreatic pseudocyst. Annals of the Royal College of Surgeons of England. 2010;**92**(1):W21-W23

[34] Johst P, Tsiotos GG, Sarr MG. Pancreatic ascites: A rare complication of necrotizing pancreatitis: A case report and review of the literature. International Journal of Pancreatology. 1997;**22**(2):151-154

[35] Bhasin DK, Malhi NS, Nagi B, Singh K. Pancreatic ascites treated by endoscopic pancreatic sphincterotomy alone: A case report. Gastrointestinal Endoscopy. 2003;**57**(6):802-804

[36] Bhandari R, Chamlagain R, Bhattarai S, Tischler EH, Mandal R, Bhandari RS. Pancreatic ascites managed with a conservative approach: A case report. Journal of Medical Case Reports. 2020;**14**(1):154

[37] Sankaran S, Sugawa C, Walt AJ. Value of endoscopic retrograde pancreatography in pancreatic ascites. Surgery, Gynecology & Obstetrics. 1979;**148**(2):185-192

[38] Soto JA, Barish MA, Yucel EK, Clarke P, Siegenberg D, Chuttani R, et al. Pancreatic duct: MR cholangiopancreatography with a three-dimensional fast spin-echo technique. Radiology. 1995;**196**(2):459-464

[39] Bresler L, Boissel P, Grosdidier J. Major hemorrhage from pseudocysts and pseudoaneurysms caused by chronic pancreatitis: Surgical therapy. World Journal of Surgery. 1991;**15**(5):649-652

[40] Yeo CJ, Bastidas JA, Lynch-Nyhan A, Fishman EK, Zinner MJ, Cameron JL. The natural history of pancreatic pseudocysts documented by computed tomography. Surgery, Gynecology & Obstetrics. 1990;**170**(5):411-417

[41] Chiang KC, Chen TH, Hsu JT. Management of chronic pancreatitis complicated with a bleeding pseudoaneurysm. World Journal of Gastroenterology. 2014;**20**(43):16132-16137

[42] Balachandra S, Siriwardena AK. Systematic appraisal of the management of the major vascular complications of pancreatitis. American Journal of Surgery. 2005;**190**(3):489-495

[43] Turnes J, García-Pagán JC, González M, Aracil C, Calleja JL, Ripoll C, et al. Portal hypertension-related complications after acute portal vein thrombosis: Impact of early anticoagulation. Clinical Gastroenterology and Hepatology. 2008;**6**(12):1412-1417

[44] Tateishi A, Mitsui H, Oki T, Morishita J, Maekawa H, Yahagi N, et al. Extensive mesenteric vein and portal vein thrombosis successfully treated by thrombolysis and anticoagulation. Journal of Gastroenterology and Hepatology. 2001;**16**(12):1429-1433

[45] Aytekin C, Boyvat F, Kurt A, Yologlu Z, Coskun M. Catheter-directed thrombolysis with transjugular access in portal vein thrombosis secondary to pancreatitis. European Journal of Radiology. 2001;**39**(2):80-82

[46] Rammohan A, Palaniappan R, Ramaswami S, Perumal SK, Lakshmanan A, Srinivasan UP, et al. ISRN Radiology. 2013;**2013**:191794

[47] Ru N, Zou WB, Qian YY, Tang XY, Zhu JH, Hu LH, et al. A systematic review of the etiology, diagnosis, and treatment of hemosuccus pancreaticus. Pancreas. 2019;**48**(5):e47-e49

[48] Renzulli P, Hostettler A, Schoepfer AM, Gloor B, Candinas D. Systematic review of atraumatic splenic rupture. The British Journal of Surgery. 2009;**96**(10):1114-1121

[49] Jain D, Lee B, Rajala M. Atraumatic splenic hemorrhage as a rare complication of pancreatitis: Case report and literature review. Clinical Endoscopy. 2020;**53**(3):311-320

[50] Hasegawa N, Ito Y, Yamaura M, Endo M, Ishige K, Fukuda K, et al. Splenic rupture caused by pancreatic pseudocyst successfully treated by endoscopic ultrasound-guided drainage. Clinical Journal of Gastroenterology. 2020;**13**(5):981-984

[51] Moori P, Nevins EJ, Wright T, Bromley C, Rado Y. A case of a chronic pancreatic pseudocyst causing atraumatic splenic rupture without evidence of acute pancreatitis. Case Reports in Surgery. 2016;**2016**:2192943

[52] Sawrey M, Hughes RG. An interesting cause of collapse in a patient with chronic pancreatitis. BML Case Reports. 2013:bcr2013009168

[53] Honda H, Miyatani H, Ikeya T, Yamanaka K, Ikeda M, Ushimaru S, et al. Endoscopic ultrasound-guided transmural cyst drainage (EUS-CD) was effective in a case of pancreatic pseudocyst with obstructive jaundice and duodenal stenosis. Nihon Shokakibyo Gakkai Zasshi. 2010;**107**(9):1497-1504

[54] Okabe Y, Tsuruta O, Wada Y, Wada K, Suga H, Kudoh M, et al. Endoscopic ultrasonography-guided cystogastrostomy for large pancreatic pseudocyst with obstructive jaundice: A case report. The Kurume Medical Journal. 2006;**53**(3-4):89-94

Section 5

Nutrinional Therapy

Chapter 8

Dietary Interventions for Pancreatitis

Mariasara Persano, Maria Lisa Marcon, Elisa Paccagnella, Claudia Vigo and Agostino Paccagnella

Abstract

Pancreatic insufficiency, both acute and chronic, is an important cause of maldigestion and malnutrition caused by impaired exocrine pancreatic function. Many causes are able to determine pancreatic insufficiency which, depending on the severity, can manifest itself with very diversified symptoms. The chapter will illustrate the diagnostic and monitoring methods of pancreatic pathology in the acute and chronic phases. Great attention will be given to oral nutrition, in its various forms, including enteral and peranterior artificial nutrition. Finally, we will discuss the most appropriate pharmacological therapy to optimise food absorption in the different phases of the disease. Each of the aspects considered takes into account the most recent literature and the clinical experience of the authors.

Keywords: acute pancreatitis, chronic pancreatitis, artificial nutrition, pancreatic insufficiency, pancreas diet

1. Introduction

1.1 Symptoms and causes of acute pancreatitis

Pancreatitis is an inflammatory process, either acute or chronic, resulting from the outset, caused by digestive enzymes, of a process of self-digestion of the pancreas, and resulting in a complex inflammatory pattern which is extremely challenging for patients. Since even organs and systems located far from the pancreas can be variably involved in such pattern, the manifestations and the intensity of the disease may prove extremely severe, to the point of endangering the patient's life [1, 2].

A healthy pancreas synthesises over 10 digestive enzymes in the acinal cells, while the pancreatic ducts host the production of bicarbonate, whose function is that of neutralising the acid content of the stomach when it reaches the duodenum. The increased pH makes the duodenum the ideal environment for the pancreatic and the jejunal digestive brush border enzymes. Complex factors contribute to the stimulation of the exocrine pancreas, including the intake of highly caloric food (>500 kcal), the presence of free fatty acids in the duodenum, the intake of essential aminoacids (phenylalanine, valine, methionine, tryptophane) and solid rather than liquid or semi-liquid dietary consumption (slower gastric emptying). The exocrine stimulation mainly occurs through the vagus nerve and the secretion of cholecystokinin (CCK) [3–5].

The onset of Acute Pancreatitis may be sudden, with pain ranging from mild to severe and often accompanied by fever, nausea and vomiting. The intensity of the pain, typically located in the epigastric area, is not always correlated with the disease severity and may radiate towards the back, the chest or the hips (**Tables 1** and **2**) [6, 7].

Data regarding the severity of the clinical picture and that of any complications are essential in the prognosis. Scores have been elaborated aimed at quantifying the severity of the clinical picture (Ranson's score; Harmless Acute Pancreatitis Score [HAPS]; Modified Glasgow Acute Pancreatitis Severity Score; Atlanta Score for Acute Pancreatitis 2013; Bedside Index for Severity in Acute Pancreatitis) [8–12]. These scores are frequently associated with systemic assessment scores such as the Marshall Score (**Table 3**) [13]. Predictive symptoms of clinical worsening in patients with Acute Pancreatitis are: body temperature < 36 o > 38°C (<96 or > 100°F), heart rate > 90/min, respiratory rate > 20/min, white blood cells <4 x 109/L or > 12 x 109 L (<4 or > 12 K/mm3).

SYMPTOMS	SIGNS
1. Pain: • generally sudden onset • mainly in the upper abdomen/epigastric area • persistent, progressively increasing intensity (not relieved by ordinary analgesics) • duration: from hours to a day • often radiated towards the back, the chest and the hips • often relieved by fetal position; 2. Associated symptoms: nausea, vomiting, anorexia, abdominal distension; 3. Aggravating factors: eating or drinking (especially alcohol); 4. Korte's sign: painful resistance in the epigastric area where the head of the pancreas is located, 6–7 cm above the navel.	1. General condition: distress, anxiety; 2. Vital signs: fever, tachycardia, hypotension, tachypnea; 3. Clinical signs: jaundice, cyanosis, dehydration 4. Abdominal pain: marked epigastric tenderness with voluntary and involuntary shielding +/− rigidity, abdominal distension, reduced peristalsis, sometimes palpable pseudocyst; 5. Possible pleural effusion; 6. Common signs associated with pancreatitis: • Voskresynskyy sign: absence of abdominal aortic pulsation in epigastric area; • Mayo-Robson sign: costovertebral angle (CVA) tenderness; • Razdolsky sign: tenderness during pancreas percussion; 7. Uncommon signs associated with severe Necrotizing Pancreatitis: • Cullen sign (presence of peri-umbilical oedema with bruising as a result of intraperitonal haemorrhage) • Grey-Turner's sign (brownish colouration of the flanks, generally between the last rib and the top of the hip, as a result of retroperitoneal haemorrhage) • Fox's sign (discolouration below the inguinal ligament or at the base of the penis) • Panniculitis, reddish skin nodules and Erythematosis (subcutaneous fat necrosis) 8. Systemic signs: • Arthritis and Sierositis resulting from the release of cytokines (a phenomenon which is not well defined from a rheumatological standpoint) • Purtscher Retinopathy (rare vasculopathy leading to sudden blindness due to retinal artery occlusion).

Table 1.
Symptoms and signs of acute pancreatitis.

Abdominal pain: 95–100%
Epigastric tenderness: 95–100%
Nausea and vomiting: 70–90%
Low-grade fever: 70–85%
Hypotension: 20–40%
Jaundice: 30%
Grey Turner/Cullen sign: <5%

Table 2.
Frequency of signs and symptoms in acute pancreatitis.

ORGAN SYSTEM	score				
	0	1	2	3	4
respiratory (PaO2/FIO2)	>400	301–400	201–300	101–200	<=101
renal (serum creatinine, mg/dL)	<1.4	1.4–1.8	1.9–3.6	3.6–4.9	>4.9
cardiovascular (systolic blood pressure, mmHg)	>90	<90	<90	<90	<90

Note: score ≥ 2 over a period of more than 48 hours, for any one of the three organ systems: persistent organ failure; score ≥ 2 over a period of less than 48 hours: transient organ failure.

Table 3.
Modified Marshall system to evaluate organ failure.

The main aetiopathological mechanisms involved in Acute Pancreatitis are summarised in **Figure 1** [14]. Their main cause is the obstruction, due to the presence of gallstones, of the biliary tract or pancreatic duct (40–70% of cases). The second

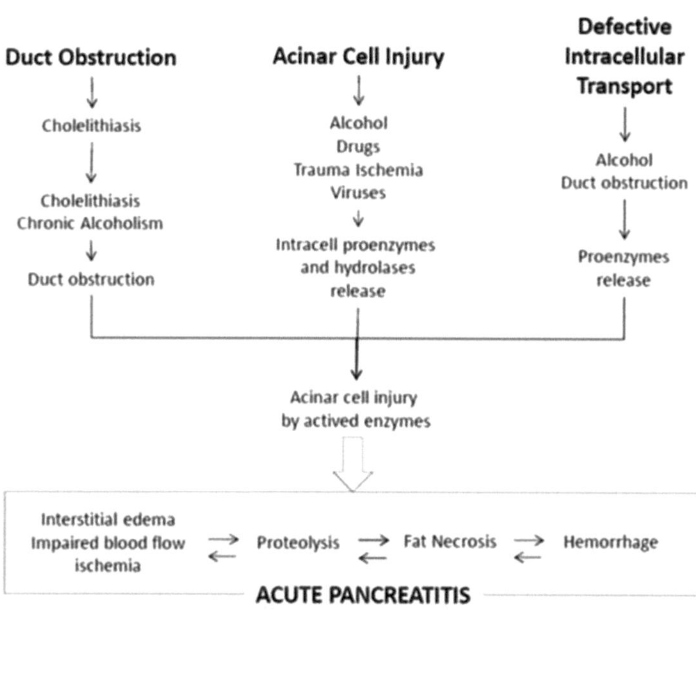

Figure 1.
Main mechanisms involved in acute pancreatitis.

• Gallstones
• Alchol (Ethanol)
• Trauma
• Cancer
• Endoscopic Retrograde Cholangiopancreatography (ERCP)
• Surgical (Post-operative)
• Mumps, Coxsackie or Idiopathic infections
• Autoimmune (Polyarteritis Nodosa)
• Genetic (Serine Protease Inhibitor Kajal Type 1), PRSS1 mutation (cationic trypsinogen)
• Hypertriglyceridemia, Hypercalcemia
• Hypothermia
• Drugs (Corticosteroids, Thiazides, Valproate, Azathioprine, Oestrogen, Sulfonamides, Tetracycline, 6-Mercaptopurine, anti-HIV medications)

Table 4.
Main causes of acute pancreatitis.

most frequent cause is alcohol consumption (25–35% of cases). Other less common causes are hyper-triglyceridemia (>1.000 mg/dL) and the presence of benign or malign Pancreatic tumours (**Table 4**). The immune system appears to play an important role in the progression of Acute Pancreatitis, since the release of pro-inflammatory mediators during the self-digestion phase might result in Necrotizing Pancreatitis. In this context, the small intestine barrier may become permeable to the transit of bacteria (bacterial translocation) from the enteric lumen to the lymphatic and blood systems, allowing Multiple Organ Dysfunction Syndrome to occur (**Figure 2**) [15, 16].

1.2 General aspects of pancreatitis treatment

Acute Pancreatitis can be classified according to clinical severity (**Table 5**) [2]. While in cases of Mild or Moderate Acute Pancreatitis organ failure and/or pancreatic necrosis hardly occur, in Medium-Severe cases there may be pancreas tissue necrosis without persistent organ failure; in severe cases, the disease progression can have an initial phase with local inflammation of the pancreas associated with a systemic inflammatory response related to the syndrome/organ failure, and a later phase with local complications and/or persistent organ damage. It is estimated that about 15–20% of the patients present a Severe Pancreatitis profile with organ failure (>8 hours). Another 20% present a Necrotizing Pancreatitis profile defined as focal areas of non-viable pancreatic parenchyma (>3 cm in size or > 30% of the pancreas) [18].

Being this distinction among Mild, Medium and Severe Pancreatitis obviously reductive and not always immediate, Acute Pancreatitis is diagnosed, in presence of abdominal pain in patients with a medical history and/or familiarity for the disease, by monitoring pancreatic health (serum amylase or lipase at least three times higher than the highest value within the normal range). Abdominal Imaging (CT or MRI) is generally crucial for the diagnosis (**Table 6**) [19, 20].

The treatment is aimed at reducing the systemic inflammatory response so as to prevent, where possible, organ failure and systemic complications. There being no

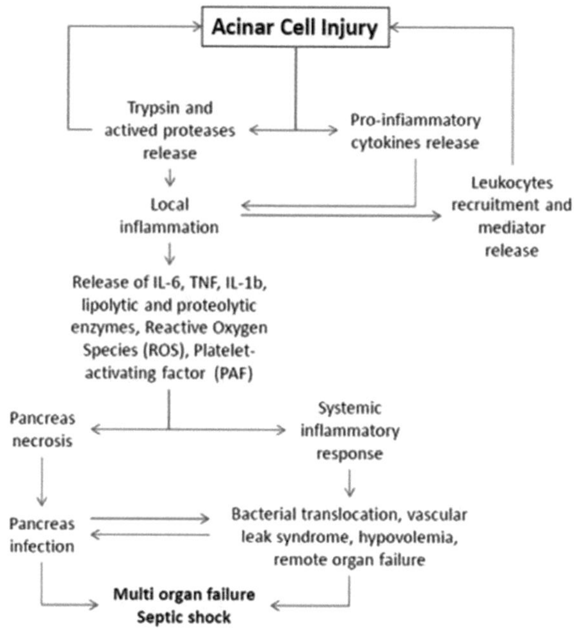

Figure 2.
Multi-organic mechanisms involved in acute pancreatitis.

Grade of Severity of Acute Pancreatitis	Criteria of Classification
Mild	No organ failure No local or systemic complications
Medium-Severe	Transient organ failure (that resolves within 48 hours) Local or systemic complications without persistent organ failure
Severe	Persistent organ failure (>48 hours) Local or systemic complications

Table 5.
Grading severity of acute pancreatitis according to Atlanta criteria 2012 [17].

• Transabdominal ultrasound should be performed in all patients with suspected Acute Pancreatitis;
• Hyper-triglyceridemia (>1.000 mg/dl), once ascertained, should be considered a major cause of the disease in the absence of gallstones and/or history of alcohol consumption/abuse;
• A neoplastic origin should always be considered in patients aged over 40 years;
• Patients with Idiopathic Pancreatitis should be re-evaluated over time and possibly sent to specialised centres;
• Genetic testing should be considered in young patients (<30 years) if there is no obvious cause or, conversely, if there is familiarity for pancreatic diseases.

Table 6.
Diagnostic aspects in patients with pancreatitis.

specific pharmacological treatment to this date, hydro-electrolyte re-balancing, use of analgesics, antibiotics and management of metabolic complications (hyperglycemia and hypocalcemia) are at the core of today's treatment.

Overall, Mild Acute Pancreatitis should be treated with fluids, analgesics and antibiotics for a few days only in presence of infectious complications (never for prophylactic purposes), whereas Severe Acute Pancreatitis requires an accurate inspection, since patients must undergo surgical removal of gallstones, re-activation of the bilious-pancreatic ducts and, in rare cases, elimination of the necrotic tissue through partial or total removal of the the pancreas and/or attached organs [21].

1.3 Evaluation of the nutritional status

Maximum catabolism with negative nitrogen balance is not uncommon, especially in the most severe cases of Acute Pancreatitis [22, 23]. The resulting high increase in calorie (Resting Energy Expenditure) and protein need might rapidly lead, if not promptly managed, to malnutrition (**Figure 3**) [24]. Malnutrition, being associated with severe weight loss, lean body mass loss and decreased functional capacity due to sarcopenia, is likely to affect quality of life and clinical outcomes [25]. Possibly asthenia and/or loss of appetite, leading to reduced calorie-protein intake, contribute to weight loss, hence to malabsorption and maldigestion. In case of sudden weight loss (10% of habitual weight in about 3–6 months), malnutrition might pair with the main disease, leading to acute or chronic complications which may worsen the patient's prognosis (**Table** 7).

Therefore, the aetiology of malnutrition is heterogeneous and may depend on the severity of the disease, the patient's ability to eat food and the catabolic state. Old age and immobilisation may contribute to raise the risk of malnutrition (**Figure 4**) [26]. Full-blown malnutrition becomes a disease which adds up to the underlying disease. Patients with Acute Pancreatitis should be considered at high risk of malnutrition.

To confirm this, literature shows that about 30% of patients with Acute Pancreatitis are malnourished and that they do not receive adequate nutritional support, which makes accurate Nutritional Screenings such as the Nutritional Risk Screening 2002 (NRS-2002) necessary in order to objectively evaluate the risk of hypo/malnutrition. **Table 8** shows some of the most employed Screening Tools.

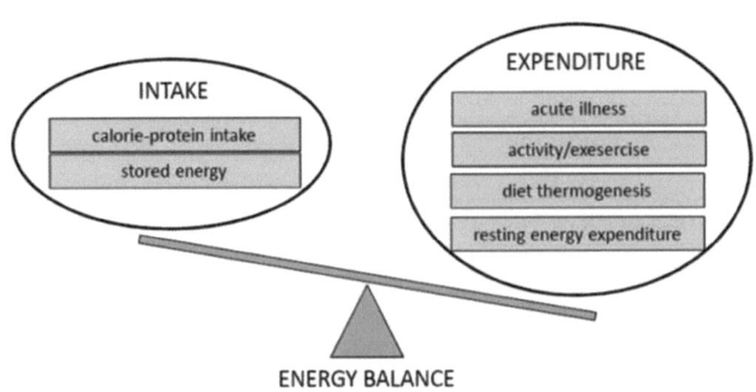

Figure 3.
Relationship between energy intake and expenditure (see text).

Short-term consequences	Long-term consequences
• Weight reduction with muscle and fat loss	• Decreased long-term survival
• Biochemical disorders (anaemia and hypoalbuminaemia)	• Risk of secondary tumours
• Late bone marrow recovery	• Higher mortality
• Changes in body composition	• Alteration of bone density and/or osteoporosis
• Immunodepression and slow wound healing	• Decreased life quality and productivity
• Increased susceptibility to infections	• Higher levels of psychological discomfort
• Longer hospitalisation stay and higher re-hospitalisation frequency	
• Increased healthcare costs	
• Decreased tolerance to chemotherapy	
• Adverse response to chemo-radio therapy	
• Delayed chemo-radio therapy	

Table 7.
Consequences of malnutrition.

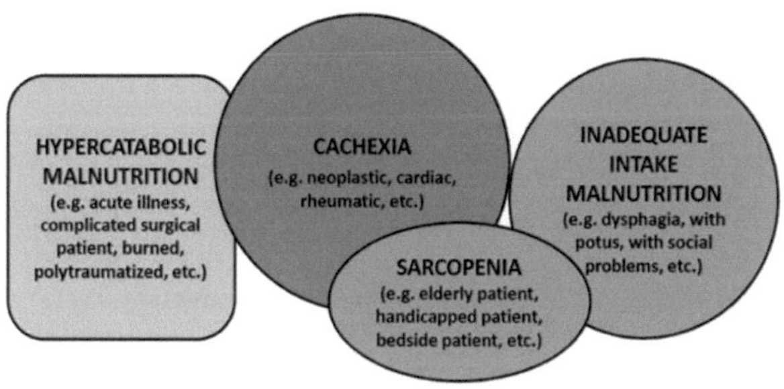

Figure 4.
A schematic overview of the different types of malnutrition.

Screening	• Malnutrition Screening Tool (MST). • Malnutrition Universal Screening Tool (MUST). • Nutritional Risk Index (NRI). • Nutrition Risk in Critically Ill (NUTRIC) score.
Diagnostic Assessment	• Subjective Global Assessment (SGA). • Patient Generated Subjective Global Assessment (PS-SGA). • Mini Nutritional Assessment (MNA). • AND (Academy of Nutrition and Dietetics)-ASPEN (American Society for Parenteral and Enteral Nutrition) Malnutrition Consensus Criteria (MCC). • Global Leadership Initiative on Malnutrition (GLIM).

Table 8.
Malnutrition screening and diagnostic assessment tools (used in the USA, Australia, New Zealand, Canada and Europe).

The employment of a Screening Tool permits to immediately evaluate the nutritional status and to monitor the progression of the disease. Unfortunately, these tools are scarcely used and patients' nutritional treatment is not adequate.

1.4 Nutritional treatment of acute pancreatitis

Acute Pancreatitis is traditionally treated with the suspension of food intake via mouth in order to rest the pancreas. This indication is suggested until pain is resolved or until the normalisation of the flogoses indices and/or until the pancreatic enzymes fall within acceptable normal values. However, the nutritional treatment should be planned and monitored over time, and it should include: (1) accurate evaluation of the severity of the disease; (2) proper assessment of the nutritional state; (3) correct identification of the patients with special nutritional needs. As shown in the previous paragraphs, Acute Pancreatitis may present itself very differently in clinic, thus requiring differentiated nutritional approaches.

1.4.1 Energy and protein need in acute pancreatitis

The Resting Energy Expenditure (REE) in patients with Acute Pancreatitis depends on the severity of the disease. In the most severe cases it is highly increased, thus entailing a high mortality risk linked to increased catabolism. In patients with septic complications the REE may be increased by decreased splanchnic blood flow, acidosis and bacterial translocation, as a result of which the REE assessed via indirect calorimetry (REEm) may exceed up to 110–150% of the energy expenditure theoretically calculated using Harris-Benedict (REEc) formulas. A realistic evaluation at the patient's bed should assess the energy expenditure by means of REEc multiplied by a constant of 1,3 or 1,5, depending on the clinical severity. As a result of this huge energy consumption, skeletal muscle proteolysis might increase up to 80% with nitrogen losses of 20–40 g per day, hence requiring the energy and the protein need to be estimated around, respectively, 25 kcal/kg/die and 1,2–1,5 g/kg/die [24, 27, 28].

1.4.2 Oral vs. artificial nutrition in moderate acute pancreatitis

Oral feeding is recommended when abdominal pain, nausea and vomiting have disappeared and, according to some authors, food intake may also take place regardless of serum lipase concentrations [29]. In this context the ideal diet includes a gradual intake of solid food and calories. Traditional diets with clear liquids and low fats (< 30% of total energy intake) have proved completely ineffective if not worsening in terms of malnutrition [30]. Early oral feeding (within 24–48 hours) should be administered also to patients undergoing minimally invasive necrosectomy, as long as haemodynamically stable, in the absence of septic complications and with normal gastro-enteric function. The use of Oral Nutritional Supplements (ONS) aimed at increasing the caloric-protein content is also recommended for these patients [31].

Being a negative prognostic factor of the disease, hyperlipaemia should be treated early with low-fat diets or, in the most severe cases, with hypolipidaemic drugs including insulin, heparin and plasmapheresis if necessary (**Figure 5**). Careful management of hyperglyceridemia appears to reduce the risk of acute pancreatitis recurrence.

Oral Nutrition has not proved less effective than Enteral Nutrition (EN) in preventing infection or death in these patients. Instead, **Table 9** shows a list of the cases in which EN after placement of nose-gastric probe is recommended.

Despite there being few data comparing it to Oral Nutrition, EN is very likely to improve these patients' prognosis, as we will see later. It should therefore be suggested early even when the development of Pancreatitis is initially uncertain (**Table 10**) [32].

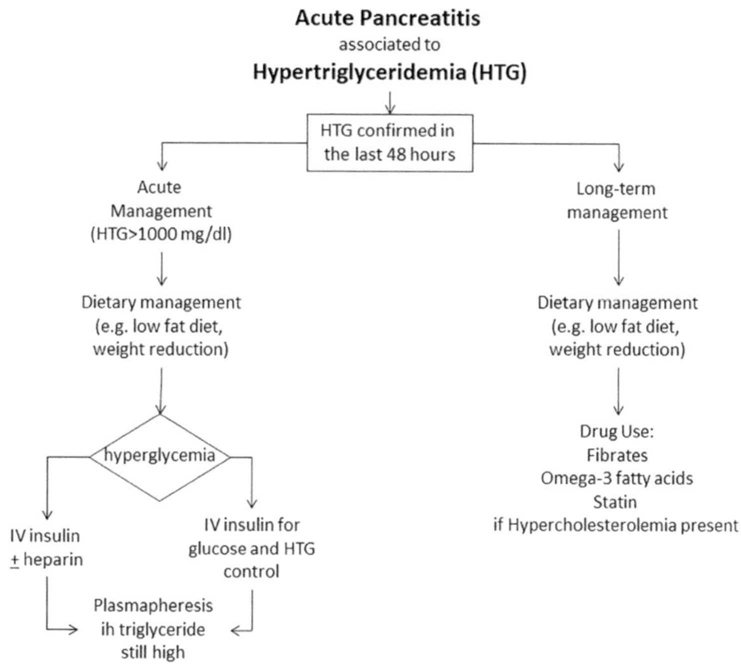

Figure 5.
Overview of management of hypertriglyceridemia.

• if Oral Nutrition is is not feasible within 24–72 hours;
• if caloric intake (also by support of Oral Supplements) does not cover at least 75% of the caloric-protein need, calculated on current weight;
• if a patient reports a rapid weight loss in the last few months (10% in the last 3–6 months);
• if Nutritional Screening strongly suggests malnutrition risk (e.g. alcohol-addicts or elderly)
• if BMI upon admission is <19 kg/m2, regardless of the clinical presentation;
• if mild painful symptoms, with nausea or vomiting, persist for a few days.

Table 9.
Indications for the use of EN during acute pancreatitis.

Nutrition Route	Pros	Cons
Oral	• No procedures or devices required • Nutrition regimen/caloric intake more easily adjustable • Easier transition to home regimen	• Increased risk of worsening Pancreatitis • Increased risk of morbidity/mortality • Wider range of variation in caloric intake day to day • Difficult to ensure adequate intake at home
Nasogastric (NG)	• Easy bedside access • No need for enteral pump • Permits higher feeding rates and bolus feeds	• Possible increased risk of pancreatic stimulation and worsening Pancreatitis • Nasal necrosis or sinusitis • Not suitable in patients with gastric outlet obstruction and/or need for gastric venting

Nutrition Route	Pros	Cons
Nasojejunal (NJ)	• Potentially reduced risk of aspiration • Permits enteral access beyond points of duodenal compression from inflamed pancreas • Possibly reduced risk of pancreatic stimulation	• Post pyloric placement may be difficult • Requires pump for feeding • Bolus feeding not possible • Increased risk of tube clogging/dislodgement • Nasal necrosis or sinusitis • May migrate back into stomach
Percutaneous Gastrostomy with Jejunal Extension (PEG-J)	• Durable enteral access • No risk of nasopharyngeal injury • Permits gastric venting in outlet obstruction • May be placed endoscopically, radiologically, surgically	• Risk associated with tube placement (bleeding, infection, perforation) • Peristomal tube leak, bleeding, infection • Relatively contra-indicated in patients with ascites, bleeding diatheses or poor window for PEG placement • J-arm may migrate back into stomach
Parenteral Nutrition (PN)	• Direct Nutrition that bypasses need for luminal absorption • Can be used for patients with bowel obstruction or perforation • Can be used for patients with intractable nausea and vomiting	• Requires peripheral/central venous access • Increased risk for line related infections and DVT vein thrombosis • Increased risk of mucosal barrier dysfunction with resultant bacterial translocation/infection • Increased morbidity/mortality compared with EN • Increase risk of hyperglycaemia

Table 10.
Pros and cons on nutrition route in severe acute pancreatitis.

1.4.3 Artificial nutrition in severe acute pancreatitis

Being the risk of malnutrition in Severe Acute Pancreatitis particularly worrying, Parenteral Nutrition (PN) has been widely considered a first choice therapy in the past, aimed at providing such a caloric-protein intake able to maintain lean mass without stimulating the pancreas [33, 34]. However, more recent data show that PN is associated with higher risk of infections (especially from the venous catheter), besides triggering electrolyte imbalance, leading to – or aggravating – Pancreatitis-induced hyperglycaemia and increasing the risk of multi-organ dysfunction. Since PN administration does not involve enteric transit, the intestinal mucosa is at risk of atrophy, with consequent reduction of its barrier function, especially in the small intestine, thus leading to bacterial translocation [35]. All these phenomena may worsen the clinical picture.

Given these considerations, EN through nose-gastric probe should be carried out early (within 24–72 hours) in haemodynamically stable patients who do not tolerate Oral Nutrition, so as to protect the intestinal mucosa, prevent the proliferation of bacteria and stimulate bowel motility (**Figure 6**) [36, 37]. Many studies and meta-analyses show that EN significantly decreases the rate of infection (with lower levels of cytotoxic CD4 T lymphocytes and C-reactive protein), the risk of multi-organ failure, the necessity for operation and the mortality, compared to PN. Gastric EN does not lead to higher incidence of complications (such as diarrhoea, abdominal distension or increased pain), although the indication to use anti-secretory agents (somatostatin, octreotide) so as to reduce the nutrients-induced secretory action of the pancreas remains questioned.

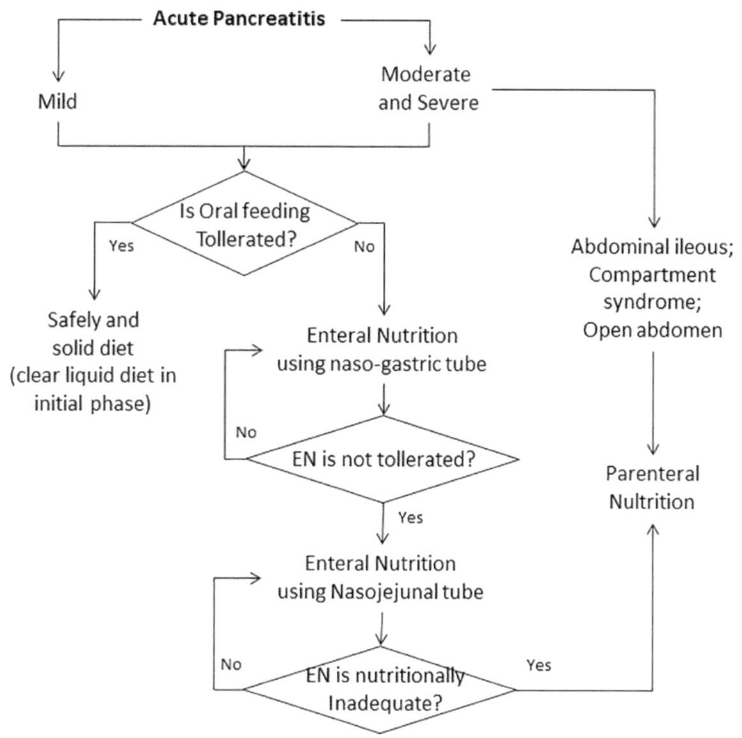

Figure 6.
Route of nutrition treatment in acute pancreatitis.

In cases where the enteric function appears uncertain, it is recommendable not to infuse nutrients, but only a 5% low-speed glucosate solution (10–20 ml/hour for 24 hours) through the standard gastric-nose probe. The evaluation of the gastric stagnation or the distension of the loops, in addition to the use of instrumental techniques, will permit to assess the state of the enteric transit. The use of a nasojejunal probe (NJ) is recommended in patients with gastroparesis, gastric obstruction due to oedema or pancreatic pseudocyst. Since the tip of this probe, which is indicated also in case of significant regurgitation, ideally overcomes the Treitz ligament, its insertion may prove difficult, often requiring repeated positioning by endoscopy and resulting in frequent spontaneous displacement. In Severe Necrotizing Pancreatitis or in Nasopharyngeal Disorder precluding NJ placement, some scholars suggest the placement of a percutaneous gastrostomy tube with jejunal extension (PEG-J) in case of EN lasting over 4–6 weeks. These invasive techniques should be used only with complicated patients in whom the prognosis appears to be severely impaired. Finally, jejunostomy should be performed in patients undergoing surgery (**Table 11**) [38].

A possible side effect of EN is the increased Intra-Abdominal Pressure (IAP), due to which the use of boluses is never recommended, especially in case the patient is feverish or reports nausea or vomiting. On the contrary, a low flow of nutrients (20 ml/hour to be increased very slowly depending on the patient's tolerance) can guarantee, especially in the early stages, a progressive normalisation of the intestinal function.

In the most severe cases, measurement of Pulmonary Pressure is recommended. When it reaches or exceeds 15 mmhg, EN should be administered with caution. In

Management of severe Pancreatitis	Nutritional Recommendations
Enteral vs. Parenteral Nutrition	Enteral preferred
Timing of feeding	Enteral feeding within 48 hours
Gastric vs. jejunual route	No difference
Oral food composition	No difference were observed using normal fat, low-fat, soft diet with liquid or solid
Enteral formula	No benefit of semi-elemental or elemental formula vs. polymeric formula
Enteral infusion	Continuous low-flow feeding (no bolus)
Probiotics use	Not recommended

Table 11.
Overall nutritional recommendations for severe acute pancreatitis.

patients with pressures above 15 mmhg, in which a picture of abdominal hypertension is possible (e.g. no peristalsis, abdominal distension, elevated gastric stagnation, etc.), the development of a picture of Abdominal Compartment Syndrome (ACS) should never be excluded [39]. In this context, the use of a nasojejunal tube for EN should be preferred, although the transition to NP should always be considered. In case of IAP with pressure higher than 20 mmhg, the use of EN should be interrupted for precautionary purposes. Clinical data are reported where early EN was possible in about 30% of cases with excellent clinical results (e.g. open abdomen with rapid fascial closure, low rates of fistulation, reduction of nosocomial infections and lower hospital costs), as long as the medical staff is highly skilled in managing minimal complications and able to monitor and manage the metabolic aspects of the disease. In summary, when nutritional objectives are not attainable with EN alone, a partial or total PN should be ensured especially in hyper-catabolic patients, patients with negative nitrogen balance, patients whose gastro-enteric tract is not usable, or for whom a surgical decompression (open abdomen) is required. In these cases the additional use of glutamine (0.20 g/kg/day) appears to increase albuminaemia, decrease C-reactive protein, reduce the frequency of infections and the risk of death [40].

The use of NP should also be recommended in patients with chylous ascites not responding to a fat-free diet nor to an elemental EN diet.

1.4.4 Enteral nutrition formulations

In patients with AP, a standard polymeric diet shall be used, although some studies express concern about the possibility for these nutritional formulations to induce insufficiency of exocrine pancreas (manifesting with alteration of faecal elastase and faecal fat) especially in cases of Alcoholic or Necrotizing Pancreatitis. However, polymeric diets should always be the first choice [41]. Feeding with semi-elemental diet should be performed only if persistent steatorrhea appears and absence of clostridium-difficile infection can be proved. In case of steatorrhea the use of pancreatic enzymes should be considered. The use of semi-elemental or elemental products is appropriate in cases where, despite the severity of the clinical picture (e.g. necrotizing pancreatitis), total or partial EN is possible [42]. The enteral formulations should be chosen according to the doses of faecal elastase. Despite there being several different techniques, EN in patients with Acute Pancreatitis is mostly performed with nasogastric probe.

2. Chronic pancreatitis

2.1 Causes and symptoms of chronic pancreatitis

Chronic Pancreatitis is a fibroinflammatory syndrome of the pancreatic gland histologically characterised by irreversible morphological changes. The evolution towards a picture of Chronic Pancreatitis usually occurs due to recurring episodes of Acute Pancreatitis with permanent organ damage [43, 44]. The use of alcohol and tobacco, as well as the chronic presence of hypercalcaemia and the use of certain drugs, may contribute to the progression of the disease (**Table 12**) [46–49]. Recent studies show the persistence of a chronic inflammation process also in Chronic Pancreatitis (with the involvement of: interleukins 4, 6, 8, 10, 12; tumour necrosis factor

Class	Examples
Toxin-metabolic	Alcohol
	Tobacco smoking
	Hypercalcemia
	Hyperlipidemia
	Chronic renal failure
	Medications
	Toxins
Idiopathic	Early onset (slower development of calcification and exocrine and endocrine insufficiency)
	Late onset (faster development of calcification and exocrine and endocrine insufficiency)
	Tropical calcific pancreatitis
Anatomical obstruction	Pancreatic divisum
	Post irradiation
Autoimmune	Autoimmune pancreatitis
Recurrent and severe acute pancreatitis	Recurrent acute pancreatitis
Genetic pancreatitis	PRSS1 mutation
	PRSS2 mutation
	CFTR mutation
	SPINK 1 mutation
	CTRC mutation
	Cationic trypsinogen mutation
	α-1 antitrypsin deficiency

CFTR, cystic fibrosis transmembrane conductance regulator; CTRC, chymotrypsin C; PRSS1, serine protease 1; PRSS2, serine protease 2; SPINK 1, serine peptidase inhibitor, Kazal type 1; TIGAR-O, Toxic-metabolic, idiopathic, genetic, autoimmune, recurrent, obstructive.

Table 12.
Causes of chronic pancreatitis by TIGAR-O classification (LIST 1 - version 2001) [45]).

[TNF-alfa]; transforming growth factor [TGF-beta]; interferon [IFN-gamma]; macrophage activity; etc.) able to increase the REE [50–52].

The prevailing symptom in over 80% of patients is epigastric pain radiating towards the column or the left upper quadrant of the abdomen [53, 54]. The pain is often postprandial and is accompanied by nausea, vomiting, diarrhoea with or without oily appearance, malodorous faeces and weight loss. However, symptoms may vary and pain might be absent in case the degenerative process affects the nerve endings. On the contrary, persisting pain might manifest in presence of the worst complications of chronic pancreatitis such as fibrosis, diabetes or tumours. A major symptom of this disease is postprandial pain, which induces a progressive reduction of the caloric-protein intake, thus leading to malnutrition, and in severe cases must be treated with opiates. Weight loss could therefore be the combined result of a progressive reduction in food intake and the increase in energy expenditure induced by chronic inflammation. Less frequent causes of chronic pancreatitis are those associated with auto-immune pathologies such as coeliac disease or inflammatory bowel diseases where, however, pain may be absent or masked by intestinal inflammation. In these patients, genetic predisposition to Pancreatitis may be proved, for example, by the presence of variants of the CFTR gene responsible for cystic fibrosis, the Serine Peptidase Inhibitor Kazal Type 1 gene (SPINK1), the Serine Protease 1 gene (PRSS1) and other genes still under study [55].

Another relevant clinical aspect is the delayed gastric emptying, perceived by a high percentage of patients. The causes of this symptom are not clear, especially in patients not undergoing surgery or not taking opioids. In patients undergoing surgery this symptom is believed to be secondary to the resection of the vagus nerve or part of the duodenum [56].

2.2 Treatment overview

The treatment of Chronic Pancreatitis is based on pain control and management of complications. In Chronic Pancreatitis, as well as in Acute Pancreatitis, it is useful to divide the clinical picture into at least three stages: a) clinical picture without complications, caused by recurring episodes of Acute Pancreatitis; b) presence of pain and local complications (pancreatic pseudocysts, calcifications and minimal involvement of adjacent organs); c) end-stage with insufficiency of exocrine and/or endocrine function (**Table 13**).

Typically, these patients will need to implement the enzyme replacement therapy and be gastro-protected with proton pump inhibitors to reduce the denaturation of

AETIOLOGY	MECHANISM
Chronic Pancreatitis, cystic fibrosis, diabetes	Altered lipase production or destruction
Pancreatic cancer	Pancreatic duct obstruction
Coeliac disease, Crohn's disease, Shwachman–Diamond syndrome	Decreased endogenous lipase stimulation and production
Gastrectomy, gastric by-pass, extensive small bowel resection	Motility disorders (interaction with chyme, decrease stimulation of pancreatic enzymes)

Table 13.
Causes of pancreatic dysfunction.

pancreatic lipase by stomach acid. The nutritional intervention, which is accompanied by hydro-electrolyte rebalancing, has proved effective not only in the prevention and treatment of malnutrition, but also in reducing the systemic inflammatory process, with reduced complications and improved prognosis of the disease.

2.3 Treatment of the endocrine insufficiency

Over 50% of patients with Chronic Pancreatitis develop Diabetes Mellitus due to mass loss of beta-cells, although Endocrine Insufficiency, which manifests in Chronic Pancreatitis, may have a double aetiology: on the one hand it is secondary to a reduced production of insulin, on the other it could depend on insulin resistance (Pancreatogenic Diabetes, or type 3 Diabetes) [57]. The diagnosis of Diabetes is obviously carried out with the same techniques used in the other types of Diabetes (fasting blood sugar dosage, load curve, C-peptide, dosage of glycosylated haemoglobin). However, the differential diagnosis is carried out by assessing the severity of the pancreatic picture and the the absence of antibodies associated with type 1 diabetes, as well as by detecting pancreatic disease via Imaging. The evaluation of the beta cell reserve function, attained by dosing a fasting C-peptide, is crucial in choosing the best drug. The treatment of patients with Pancreatogenic Diabetes could be more complex than those with type 2 Diabetes due to the concomitant presence of malabsorption, impaired secretion of counter-regulatory hormones and potential lack of compliance in the case of alchol-induced Pancreatopathy. Furthermore, the use of many antidiabetic agents is often contraindicated. There are not randomised clinical trials on hypoglycaemic treatment for diabetes associated with pancreatic disease. In case of preserved beta cell function, metformin is the first choice treatment. Side effects as nausea, weight loss, diarrhoea or the increased risk of lactic acidosis should be carefully assessed and metformin stopped if present. The use of DPP4-inhibitors or GLP1-receptor agonists is not recommended due to the reportedly increased risk of worsening the pancreatic disease.

The use of sulfonylureas as a front-line therapy is not recommended due to both the increased risk of hypoglycaemia and the dependence of intact islet cell function. Also the use of thiazolidinediones is discouraged because of their side effects (weight gain, fluid retention) and their role in increasing the risk of osteoporosis, especially in patients with calcium malabsorption. Given the progressive impairment of insulin secretion, insulin therapy with rapid and basal analogues is frequently required. Insulin therapy should be initiated without delay in case of: symptomatic hyperglycaemia (>180 mg/dl), catabolic state secondary to uncontrolled diabetes, history of diabetic keto-acidosis, hospitalisation for uncontrolled diabetes. Special attention must be paid to the management of hypoglycaemia and the gradual adjustment of insulin dose, as these patients are more likely to be insulin sensitive and to present a loss of counter regulatory hormones. Other important factors are hepatic glycogen storage deficit, carbohydrate malabsorption and malnutrition, inconsistent eating patterns due to pain or nausea, and possibly underlying alcoholic liver disease and enhanced peripheral insulin sensitivity. Diabetic education or glucose self-monitoring and glucagon utilisation should be provided to all patients. A valid alternative to capillary glycaemic control is the use of continuous or flash glucose monitoring. There are currently no studies available comparing glycaemic control in patients with pancreatic disease using self glucose blood monitoring and flash/continuous glucose monitoring. Lifestyle modifications, such as stopping smoking and drinking alcohol, are essential to reduce the risk of recurrence, since alcohol and tobacco smoking contribute to keeping the inflammatory process high, thus favouring the risk of pancreatic cancer and diabetes [58].

2.4 Nutritional assessment in chronic pancreatitis

A reduced exocrine function, especially if under-diagnosed, may on its own induce a state of hypo- or malnutrition, possibly secondary to a malabsorption of macro and micro-nutrients [59]. It is estimated that a picture of pancreatic dysfunction develops in about ten years in patients with potus and in about 20 years in those with idiopathic aetiology and that it is extremely frequent in people with autoimmune diseases. Enteric symptoms (malabsorption, bloating, diarrhoea, steatorrhea, weight loss, abdominal discomfort) are usually present when enzymatic secretion is 10% lower than normal. Since this situation is mainly linked to inadequate lipid digestion, it may result in a malabsorption of fat-soluble vitamins (vit. A: 1–16% of cases; vit. D: 33–87%; vit. E: 2–27%; vit. K: 13–63%), with loss of micro-nutrients and reduction of circulating lipoproteins (**Table 14**) [60]. In Severe Chronic Pancreatitis, the use of parenteral fat-soluble vitamins is absolutely indicated. Much less frequent is the lack of hydro-soluble vitamins with the exception of thiamine (vit. B1), which is often deficient in alcoholics. A shortage of zinc, copper and selenium has also been observed in patients who do not consume alcohol, so the use of specific supplements is recommended by a number of scholars.

The state of chronic inflammation, also variably present in Chronic Pancreatitis, can interfere with the protein synthesis and catabolism by the body. Insufficient levels of pancreatic protease may lead to protein malnutrition and be a cause of vitamin B12 deficiency. The absorption of vitamin D, calcium and folic acid, whose deficiency causes significant changes in the clinical picture, requires a separate discussion. In fact, a picture of osteopathy (osteoporosis, osteomalacia, osteopenia) is present in about a quarter of patients with Chronic Pancreatitis. Vitamin D deficiency, which is often underestimated, may present itself with not clearly defined bone pain and may trigger other diseases (**Table 15**) [61]. However, hyper-secretion of the parathyroid hormone (PTH) may be one of the first signs of vitamin D deficiency. Densitometric studies (dual-energy x-ray absorptiometry) should always be implemented to prevent or monitor any skeletal damage. Exocrine pancreas dysfunction requires a change in lifestyle (e.g. no smoking, no alcohol) and the intake of pancreatic enzymes during meals in order to reduce the effects of malabsorption-induced malnutrition. A supplementation of protein or macro-nutrients should be recommended particularly to patients who reduce their food intake or undertake unbalanced low-calorie and low-protein diets because of pain or fear of pain. Early enzymatic and vitamin supplementation should be associated with careful clinical evaluation over time.

VITAMIN	SOURCES	MAIN FUNCTIONS	DEFICIENCY
A (retinol)	fish liver oil, milk, cheese, eggs, carrots, apricots, broad-leaved vegetables	Precursor of rhodopsin, protective antitumoural action	Visual impairment, increased cancer incidence
D (cholecalciferol)	fish liver oil, eggs, milk, oily fish	Regulation of the metabolism of calcium	Rickets in children, osteomalacia in adults
E (tocopherol)	broad-leaved vegetables, oily seeds and fruits, liver, eggs, dairy products	Lipid protection from oxidation (antioxidant effect), anticancer, anti-sclerotic, additive	Accumulation of lipid peroxides, anaemia, chronic-degenerative diseases
K	Intestinal flora, vegetables	Prothrombin activation, calcium metabolism	Haemorrhages

Table 14.
Dietary sources and functions of fat-soluble vitamins.

APPARATE	DISEASE
Neuropsychiatric diseases	Schizophrenia Major depressive disorders Neurodegenerative disorders
Infections	Respiratory infections Covid-19 Sepsis Tuberculosis
Vascular diseases	Hypertension Cardiovascular diseases
Muscular diseases	Muscle pain Proximal muscle weakness
Bone diseases	Osteoporosis Osteomalacia Osteopenia Osteoarthritis
Skin diseases	Epidermolytic ichthyosis Autosomal recessive congenital ichthyosis
Allergic diseases	Asthma Wheezing diseases Urticaria Atopic dermatitis
Autoimmune diseases	Type 1 diabetes Rheumatoid arthritis Inflammatory bowel diseases Multiple sclerosis Psoriasis Vitiligo
Cancer	Breast Colon Prostate

Table 15.
Diseases secondary to vitamin D deficiency.

Figure 7 summarises the essential components of an adequate nutritional assessment [62]. If malnutrition develops, the symptoms described in **Table 5**, often blurred, or simply vitamin deficiency signs may be present. Although sarcopenia has been poorly studied in patients with Chronic Pancreatitis, it may, as in neoplastic patients, increase the risk of complications and hospitalisation. An accurate nutritional assessment is therefore always appropriate in patients with Chronic Pancreatitis.

2.5 Nutritional requirements in chronic pancreatitis

2.5.1 Oral nutrition

Low-fat oral diets are widely used in clinical practice especially for the purpose of reducing postprandial abdominal pain. However, these diets, in addition to being poorly accepted by patients, can induce a state of malnutrition [63]. In fact, it is estimated that a patient with Chronic Pancreatitis has a REE 30–50% higher than healthy patients. As an indication, diets with high energy (35 kcal/kg/24 hours), high

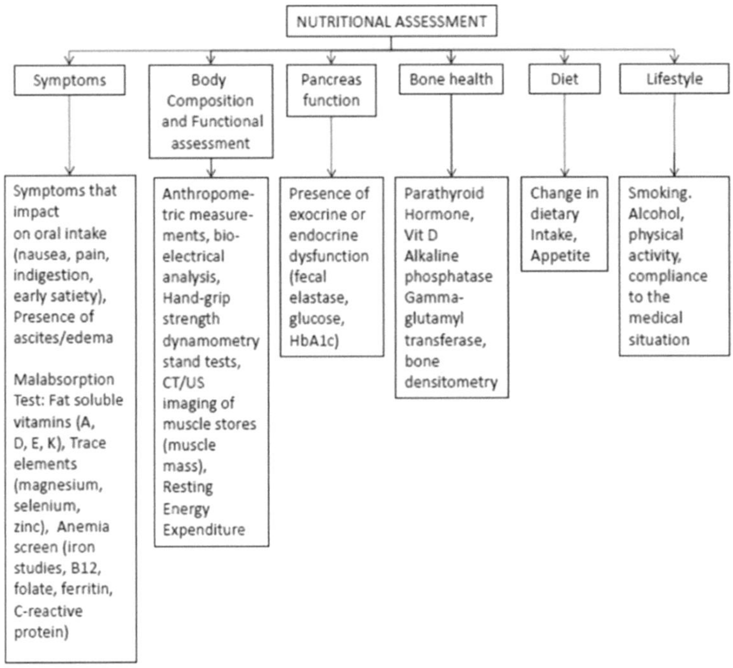

Figure 7.
Nutritional assessment in chronic pancreatitis.

protein (1.0 to 1.5 g/kg/24 hours), rich in carbohydrates, and with moderate amounts of fat (0.7 to 1.0 g/kg/24 hours) should be recommended. Low-fat diets are discouraged by a number of scholars, since they may reduce steatorrhea, thus masking the onset of fat malabsorption, induce a weight loss due to insufficient caloric intake and cause deficiencies in fat-soluble vitamins. Fats should be limited if it is not possible to control steatorrhea (generally associated with flatulence, bloating, dyspepsia, urgency to pass stools, cramping, abdominal pain) with proper oral Pancreatic Enzyme Replacement Therapy (PERT). Typically, 500 units/lipase/kg are recommended for each meal and adapted to the symptoms or the type of diet recommended for the patient. The dose can be doubled or even tripled but should never exceed 10,000 units/kg/day or 4000 units/g of fat per day [64].

In some circumstances (i.e: mixture of enzymes with meal; gastric emptying with meal; rapid release of enzymes in duodenum by chyme and bile acids) enzymatic supplementation appears scarcely effective, so it is necessary to accurately educate patients to use these products according to the quality of food intake, to its rate of intake, to its distribution and time of consumption. Benefits have also been observed by combining these therapies with antagonist H2 drugs or Proton pump inhibitor to prevent enzymatic degradation [65, 66]. To counteract the patient's weight loss, a supplementation of medium-chain triglycerides (MCT) that are absorbed in the absence of lipases, co-lipases, and bile salts is also suggested in combination with increased caloric intake. However, their use is limited by their poor palatability and the possibility of prescribing them up to a maximum of 50 g/day. Higher dosages may induce ketogenesis and intestinal disorders (cramps, nausea, diarrhoea). MCTs are found in coconut oils or in the form of oral supplements. In Chronic Pancreatitis carbohydrates and proteins should not be limited. Only in case of Diabetes should the proportion of carbohydrates, which will be balanced according to the hypoglycaemic therapy, be evaluated. A number of scholars recommend high-calorie and high-protein diets, divided into five or six small meals throughout the day, and discourage diets very rich in fibres, being fibres able to absorb or block the action of pancreatic lipase, thus modifying the absorption of nutrients, due to a still poorly known mechanism. Pancreatic enzymes are thought to be possibly absorbed or trapped by fibres and be inactivated by anti-nutrient compounds present in some foods (i.e.: aponins, trypsin end lectins in soybeans; lectins and trypsin inhibitors in legumes; polyphenols in extracts of citrus fruits, Grape seeds, tea, peanut shells and apples). Finally, it is worth remembering that in about 10% of patients the use of caloric-protein supplementation by means of oral nutritional supplements enriched with micro-nutrients and vitamins in order to prevent a significant weight loss is recommended before considering artificial nutrition treatment of enteral or parenteral type. In patients with hyperglycaemia, the treatment is similar to that described for Acute Pancreatitis. In case of preserved beta cell function, metformin is the first choice treatment also in Chronic Pancreatitis. Given the higher risk of pancreatic tumour in patients with Chronic Pancreatitis and Diabetes, the choice of metformin is further supported by its anti-neoplastic effect. Data on SGLT2-inhibitors use in Chronic Pancreatitis are still controversial; since this class of drugs could increase the risk of euglycaemic ketoacidosis in insulin-deficient patients and induce catabolic effects and dehydratation, it should be used with caution.

2.5.2 Enteral nutrition or parenteral nutrition

It is estimated that 5% of patients must regularly undergo EN to prevent or reduce malnutrition [67]. The indications for acute pancreatitis summarised in the **Table 9** also apply to Chronic Pancreatitis. Fibres should similarly be reduced to avoid interference with pancreatic enzymes.

Finally, it is estimated that only 1% of patients with Chronic Pancreatitis undergo Parenteral Nutritional treatment. Usually this treatment is reserved to patients with stenotic complications or enteric fistulas waiting for surgery.

Author details

Mariasara Persano[1], Maria Lisa Marcon[1], Elisa Paccagnella[2], Claudia Vigo[1] and Agostino Paccagnella[1]*

1 UOC di Malattie Endocrine, del Ricambio e Nutrizione, Treviso Hospital, Italy

2 UOC di Genetica Medica, Ospedale Burlo Garafalo, Trieste, Italy

*Address all correspondence to: agostino.paccagnella@aulss2.veneto.it

References

[1] Crockett SD, Wani S, Gardner TB, et al. American Gastroenterological Association Institute guideline on initial management of acute pancreatitis. Gastroenterology. 2018;**154**:1096-1101. DOI: 10.1053/j.gastro. 2018.01.032

[2] Jablonska B, Mrowiec S. Nutritional support in patients with severe acute pancreatitis-current standards. Nutrients. 2021;**13**:1498. DOI: 10.3390/ nu13051498

[3] Singh VK, Bollen TL, Wu BU, et al. An assessment of the severity of interstitial pancreatitis. Clin Gastroent Hepatol. 2011;**9**:1098-1103. DOI: 10.1016/j.cgh.2011.08.026

[4] Fusco R, Cordaro M, Siracusa R, et al. Biochemical evaluation of the antioxidant effects of hydroxytyrosol on pancreatitis-associated gut injury. Antioxidants. 2020;**9**:781. DOI: 10.3390/ antiox9090781

[5] Weiss FU, Laemmerhirt F, Lerch MM. Etiology and risk factors of acute and chronic pancreatitis. Visc Med. 2019;**35**:73-81. DOI: 10.1159/ 000499138

[6] Marik PE, Zaloga GP. Meta-analysis of parenteral nutrition versus enteral nutrition in patients with acute pancreatitis. BMJ. 2004;**328**:1407. DOI: 10.1136/bmj.38118.593900.55

[7] Pan LL, Li J, Shamoon M, et al. Recent advances on nutrition in treatment of acute pancreatitis. Frontiers in Immunology. 2017;**8**:762. DOI: 10.3389/ fimmu.2017.00762

[8] Ranson JH. Acute pancreatitis. Current Problems in Surgery. 1979;**16**: 1-84. DOI: 10.1016/s0011-3840(79) 80012-x

[9] Lankisch PG, Weber-Dany B, Hebel K, et al. The harmless acute pancreatitis score: A clinical algorithm for rapid initial stratification of nonsevere disease. Clinical Gastroenterology and Hepatology. 2009;**7**:702-705. DOI: 10.1016/j. cgh.2009.02.020

[10] Corfield AP, Cooper MJ, Williamson RC, et al. Prediction of severity in acute pancreatitis: Prospective comparison of three prognostic indices. Lancet. 1985;**2**: 403-407. DOI: 10.1016/s0140-6736(85) 92733-3

[11] Park JY, Jeon TJ, Ha TH, et al. Bedside index for severity in acute pancreatitis: Comparison with other scoring systems in predicting severity and organ failure. Hepatobiliary & Pancreatic Diseases International. 2013; **12**:645-650. DOI: 10.1016/s1499-3872 (13)60101-0

[12] Probst P, Haller S, Bruckner T, et al. Prospective trial to evaluate the prognostic value of different nutritional assessment scores in pancreatic surgery (NURIMAS pancreas). The British Journal of Surgery. 2017;**104**:1053-1062. DOI: 10.1002/bjs.10525

[13] Marshall JC, Cook DJ, Christou NV, et al. Multiple organ dysfunction score: A reliable descriptor of a complex clinical outcome. Critical Care Medicine. 1995; **23**:1638-1652

[14] Alkareemy EAR, Ahmed LAW, El-Masry MA, et al. Etiology, clinical characteristics, and outcomes of acute pancreatitis in patients at Assiut university hospital. Egypt. Journal of Internal Medicine. 2020;**32**:24. DOI: 10.1186/s43162-020-00025-w

[15] Steinberg W, Tenner S. Acute pancreatitis. The New England Journal of Medicine. 1994;**330**:1198-1210. DOI: 10.1056/NEJM199404283301706

[16] Yadav D. Recent advances in the epidemiology of alcoholic pancreatitis. Current Gastroenterology Reports. 2011; **13**:157-165. DOI: 10.1007/s11894-011-0177-9

[17] Banks PA, Bollen TL, Dervenis C, Gooszen HG, Johnson CD, Sarr MG, et al. Acute pancreatitis classification working group. Classification of acute pancreatitis–2012: Revision of the Atlanta classification and definitions by international consensus. Gut. 2013;**62**: 102-111. DOI: 10.1136/gutjnl-2012-302779

[18] Ferreira Ade F, Bartelega JA, Urbano HC, de Souza IK. Acute pancreatitis gravity predictive factors: Which and when to use them? Arquivos Brasileiros de Cirurgia Digestiva. 2015; **28**:207-211. DOI: 10.1590/S0102-67202015000300016

[19] Balthazar EJ, Robinson DL, Megibow AJ, et al. Acute pancreatitis: Value of CT in establishing prognosis. Radiology. 1990;**174**:331-336

[20] Shinagare AB, Ip IK, Raja AS, et al. Use of CT and MRI in emergency department patients with acute pancreatitis. Abdom Imaging Abdominal Imaging. 2014;**40**(2):272-277. DOI: 10.1007/s00261-014-0210-1

[21] Olson E, Perelman A, Birk JW. Acute management of pancreatitis: The key to best outcomes. Postgraduate Medical Journal. 2019;**95**:1-6. DOI: 10.1136/postgradmedj-2018-136034

[22] Ramanathan M, Aadam AA. Nutrition management in acute pancreatitis. Nutrition in Clinical Practice. 2019;**34**:S7-S12. DOI: 10.1002/ncp.10386

[23] Lakananurak N, Gramlich L. Nutrition management in acute pancreatitis: Clinical practice consideration. World Journal of Clinical Cases. 2020;**8**:1561-1573. DOI: 10.12998/wjcc.v8.i9.1561

[24] Dickerson RN, Vehe KL, Mullen JL, Feurer ID, et al. Resting energy expenditure in patients with pancreatitis. Critical Care Medicine. 1991;**19**:484-490. DOI: 10.1097/00003246-199104000-00005

[25] Gatta A, Verardo A, Bolognesi M. Hypoalbuminemia. Internal and Emergency Medicine. 2012;7:S193-S199. DOI: 10.1007/s11739-012-0802-0

[26] Baeza-Zapata AA, García-Compeán D, Jaquez-Quintana JO, et al. Acute pancreatitis in elderly patients. Gastroenterology. 2021;**161**:1736-1740. DOI: 10.1053/j.gastro.2021.06.081

[27] Bouffard YH, Delafosse BX, Annat GJ, et al. Energy expenditure during severe acute pancreatitis. JPEN Journal of Parenteral and Enteral Nutrition. 1989;**13**:26-29. DOI: 10.1177/014860718901300126

[28] Hill GL, Jonathan E: Rhoads Lecture. Body composition research: Implications for the practice of clinical nutrition. JPEN Journal of Parenteral and Enteral Nutrition. 1992;**16**:197. DOI: 10.1177/0148607192016003197

[29] Bakker OJ, van Brunschot S, van Santvoort HC, et al. Early versus on-demand Nasoenteric tube feeding in acute pancreatitis. The New England Journal of Medicine. 2014;**371**:1983-1993. DOI: 10.1056/NEJMoa1404393

[30] Sathiaraj E, Murthy S, Mansard MJ, et al. Clinical trial: Oral feeding with a

soft diet compared with clear liquid diet as initial meal in mild acute pancreatitis. Alimentary Pharmacology & Therapeutics. 2008;**28**:777-781. DOI: 10.1111/j.1365-2036.2008.03794.x

[31] Doley RP, Yadav TD, Wig JD, et al. Enteral nutrition in severe acute pancreatitis. Journal of the Pancreas: JOP. 2009;**10**:157-162

[32] Wu P, Li L, Sun W. Efficacy comparisons of enteral nutrition and parenteral nutrition in patients with severe acute pancreatitis: A meta-analysis from randomized controlled trials. Bioscience Reports. 2018;**38**. DOI: 10.1042/BSR20181515

[33] Mirtallo J, Canada T, Johnson D, et al. Task force for the revision of safe practices for parenteral nutrition. Safe practices for parenteral nutrition. JPEN Journal of Parenteral and Enteral Nutrition. 2004;**28**:S39-S70. DOI: 10.1177/0148607104028006S39

[34] Jaber S, Garnier M, Asehnoune K, et al. Anaesth Crit Care Pain Med. 2022; **41**:101060. DOI: 10.1016/j.accpm.2022.101060

[35] Kalfarentzos F, Kehagias J, Mead N, et al. Enteral nutrition is superior to parenteral nutrition in severe acute pancreatitis: Results of a randomized prospective trial. The British Journal of Surgery. 1997;**84**:1665-1669. DOI: 10.1046/j.1365-2168.1997.02851.x

[36] Li JY, Yu T. Chen GCet al: Enteral nutrition within 48 hours of admission improves clinical outcomes of acute pancreatitis by reducing complications: A meta-analysis. PLoS One. 2013;**8**: e64926. DOI: 10.1371/journal.pone.006

[37] Petrov MS, van Santvoort HC, Besselink MG, et al. Enteral nutrition and the risk of mortality and infectious complications in patients with severe acute pancreatitis: A meta-analysis of randomized trials. Archives of Surgery. 2008;**143**:1111-1117. DOI: 10.1001/archsurg.143.11.1111

[38] Chang YS, Fu HQ, Xiao YM, Liu JC. Nasogastric or nasojejunal feeding in predicted severe acute pancreatitis: A meta-analysis. Critical Care. 2013;**17**: R118. DOI: 10.1186/cc12790

[39] Smit M, Buddingh KT, Bosma B, et al. Abdominal compartment syndrome and intra-abdominal ischemia in patients with severe acute pancreatitis. World Journal of Surgery. 2016;**40**:1454e61. DOI: 10.1007/s00268-015-3388-7

[40] Dong S, Zhao Z, Li X, et al. Efficacy of glutamine in treating severe acute pancreatitis: A systematic review and meta-analysis. Frontiers in Nutrition. 2022;**9**:865102. DOI: 10.3389/fnut.2022.865102

[41] Endo A, Shiraishi A, Fushimi K, et al. Comparative effectiveness of elemental formula in the early enteral nutrition management of acute pancreatitis: A retrospective cohort study. Annals of Intensive Care. 2018;**8**:69. DOI: 10.1186/s13613-018-0414-6

[42] Petrov MS, Loveday BP, Pylypchuk RD, et al. Systematic review and meta-analysis of enteral nutrition formulations in acute pancreatitis. The British Journal of Surgery. 2009;**96**: 1243-1252. DOI: 10.1002/bjs.6862

[43] Kunovsky L, Díte P, Jabandžiev P, et al. Causes of exocrine pancreatic insufficiency other than chronic pancreatitis. Journal of Clinical Medicine. 2021;**10**:5779. DOI: 10.3390/jcm10245779

[44] Machicado JD, Yadav D. Epidemiology of recurrent acute and

chronic pancreatitis: Similarities and differences. Digestive Diseases and Sciences. 2017;**62**:1683-1691. DOI: 10.1007/s10620-017-4510-5

[45] Whitcomb DC, The North American Pancreatitis Study Group. Pancreatitis: TIGAR-O version 2 risk/etiology checklist with topic reviews, updates, and use primers. Clin Translational Gastroent. 2019;**10**: e-00027. DOI: 10.14309/ctg.0000000000000027

[46] Singh VK, Haupt ME, Geller DE, Hall JA, Diez PMQ. Less common etiologies of exocrine pancreatic insufficiency. World Journal of Gastroenterology. 2017;**23**:7059-7076. DOI: 10.3748/wjg.v23.i39.7059

[47] Lindkvist B. Diagnosis and treatment of pancreatic exocrine insufficiency. World Journal of Gastroenterology. 2013;**19**:7258-7266. DOI: 10.3748/wjg.v19.i42.7258

[48] Uc A, Fishman DS. Pancreatic disorders. Pediatric Clinics of North America. 2017;**64**:685-706. DOI: 10.1016/j.pcl.2017.01.010

[49] Pandol SJ, Gorelick FS, Gerloff A, et al. Alcohol abuse, endoplasmic reticulum stress and pancreatitis. Digestive Diseases. 2010;**28**:776-782. DOI: 10.1159/000327212

[50] Rasch S, Valantiene I, Mickevicius A, et al. Chronic pancreatitis: Do serum biomarkers provide an association with an inflammageing phenotype? Pancreatology. 2016;**16**:708-714. DOI: 10.1016/j.pan.2016.08.004

[51] Robinson SM, Rasch S, Beer S, et al. Systemic inflammation contributes to impairment of quality of life in chronic pancreatitis. Scientific Reports. 2019;**9**: 7318. DOI: 10.1038%2Fs41598-019-43846-8

[52] O'Brien SJ, Omer E, et al. Chronic pancreatitis and nutrition therapy. Nutrition in Clinical Practice. 2019;**34**: S13-S26. DOI: 10.1002/ncp.10379

[53] Ammann RW, Muellhaupt B. The natural history of pain in alcoholic chronic pancreatitis. Gastroenterology. 1999;**116**:1132-1140

[54] Fasanella KE, Davis B, Lyons J, et al. Pain in chronic pancreatitis and pancreatic cancer. Gastroenterology Clinics of North America. 2007;**36**:335-64, ix. DOI: 10.1016/j.gtc.2007.03.011

[55] Pham A, Forsmark C. Chronic pancreatitis: Review and update of etiology, risk factors, and management. F1000Res. 2018;**7**:F1000 Faculty Rev. DOI: 10.12688/f1000research.12852.1

[56] Gianotti L, Besselink MG, Sandini M, et al. Nutritional support and therapy in pancreatic surgery: A position paper of the international study group on pancreatic surgery (ISGPS). Surgery. 2018;**164**:1035-1048

[57] Ewald N, Kaufmann C, Raspe A, et al. Prevalence of diabetes mellitus secondary to pancreatic diseases (type 3c). Diabetes/Metabolism Research and Reviews. 2012;**28**:338-342. DOI: 10.1002/dmrr.2260

[58] Yadav D, Hawes RH, Brand RE, et al. Alcohol consumption, cigarette smoking, and the risk of recurrent acute and chronic pancreatitis. Archives of Internal Medicine. 2009;**169**:1035-1045

[59] Rasmussen HH, Irtun Ø, Olesen SS, et al. Nutrition in chronic pancreatitis. World Journal of Gastroenterology. 2013;**19**:7267-7275. DOI: 10.3748/wjg.v19.i42.7267

[60] Bhardwaj P, Thareja S, Prakash S, Saraya A. Micronutrient antioxidant intake in patients with chronic pancreatitis. Gastroenterol. 2004;**25**:69-72

[61] Reid IR. What diseases are causally linked to vitamin D deficiency? Arch Dis Childhood. 2016;**101**:185-189. DOI: 10.1136/archdischild-2014-307961

[62] Plewka M, Rysz J, Kujawski K. Nutrition and malnutrition in chronic pancreatitis. J Food Sci Tech. 2018;**3**: 431-439. DOI: 10.25177/JFST.3.5.4

[63] Duggan SN, Smyth ND, O'Sullivan M, et al. The prevalence of malnutrition and fat-soluble vitamin deficiencies in chronic pancreatitis. Nutrition in Clinical Practice. 2014;**29**:348-354. DOI: 10.1177/0884533614528361

[64] de la Iglesia-García D, Huang W, Szatmary P, et al. NIHR pancreas biomedical research unit patient advisory group 1; efficacy of pancre-atic enzyme replacement therapy in chronic pancre-atitis: Systematic review and meta-analysis. Gut. 2017;**66**:1354-1355. DOI: 10.1136/gutjnl-2016-312529

[65] Imrie CW, Connett G, Hall RI, Charnley RM. Review article: Enzyme supplementation in cystic fibrosis, chronic pancreatitis, pancreatic and periampullary cancer. Alimentary Pharmacology & Therapeutics. 2010;**32**: 1S-25S. DOI: 10.1111/j.1365-2036.2010.04437.x

[66] Bruno MJ, Rauws EA, Hoek FJ, Tytgat GN. Comparative effects of adjuvant cimetidine and omeprazole during pancreatic enzyme replacement therapy. Digestive Diseases and Sciences. 1994;**39**:988-992. DOI: 10.1007/BF02087549

[67] Skipworth JR, Raptis DA, Wijesuriya S, et al. The use of nasojejunal nutrition in patients with chronic pancreatitis. Journal of the Pancreas: JOP. 2011;**12**:574-580

Chapter 9

Advances in Nutritional Therapy of Acute Pancreatitis

Mariana Chávez-Tostado, Karla Verónica Chávez-Tostado, Clotilde Fuentes-Orozco, Alejandro González-Ojeda, María Luisa Mendoza-Magaña, Mario Alberto Ramírez-Herrera, Gabino Cervantes-Guevara, Guillermo Alonso Cervantes-Cardona, Enrique Cervantes-Pérez, Diana Mercedes Hernández-Corona, Tonatiuh González-Heredia, Miriam Méndez-del Villar, María Fernanda Isadora Meraz-Corona, Milton Omar Guzmán-Ornelas, Abraham Alberto Ramírez-Mendoza and Steffany Arandeni Ramírez-Mendoza

Abstract

Acute pancreatitis (AP) is a frequent abdominal acute inflammatory disorder and the leading cause of hospital admissions in gastrointestinal units. Clinical manifestations of AP vary from a mild edematous form to severe fulminant pancreatitis with major devastating complications. To date, experimental therapeutic agents remain scarce for the treatment of this disease. Nutritional therapy with appropriate nutrient supplementation is key to limiting the acute inflammation and preventing and managing complications associated with AP. This chapter focuses on novel therapeutic agents for nutritional intervention including enteral versus parenteral nutrition strategies, and nutritional supplements such as probiotics, glutamine, omega-3 fatty acids, and vitamins in the treatment of AP.

Keywords: nutritional support, nutritional supplements, acute pancreatitis, antioxidants, nutritional therapy

1. Introduction

Acute pancreatitis (AP) is defined by an inflammation of the pancreas, where several organs and other systems are involved with a potential immune response in a severe course [1] with a consecutive augmented release of hydrolytic enzymes, cytokines, and toxins, which may result in failure of several systems. Hypermetabolism is observed with a negative nitrogen balance and also augmented metabolism [2–6]. Global incidence of AP ranges from 13 to 45 cases per 100,000 population with a global estimate of 33.74 cases per 100,000 population, causing an uneven burden across the globe. Gallstones (40%–70%) and alcohol (25%–35%) are two of the most common etiologies [7–10]. AP occurs frequently with a mild clinical course. However, when necrotizing pancreatitis is observed, mortality rises up to 15% of cases [11]. When infection of pancreatic necrosis is present, organ failure or both, mortality rises to 30% [12]. Also, severe pancreatitis can cause sustained hyperglycemia, producing diabetes [13, 14]. Interventions (i.e., surgical, endoscopic, and radiological) are frequently used in some patients with AP [15], requiring nutritional support [6].

Clinical therapy in AP differs according to the severity of the disease. Therefore, adequate identification of patients with mild, moderate, or severe AP (SAP), who need nutritional support, is of great importance. Atlanta classification authors defined and stratified the severity of AP [16]: Mild AP is described with absence of organ failure or local complications; moderate-severe AP with transient organ failure and/or local complications; and SAP when persistent organ failure is observed with more than 48 hours, which usually have an ominous prognosis [16]. The first step of the clinical approach of AP consists of close monitoring of vital signs, general support with vigorous fluid resuscitation, pain relief, nutrition, correction of metabolic disorders, identification of complications, and prevention of recurrence [17]. Most of the patients have a mild course of the disease with good prognosis in most cases, but near 15% of cases develop complications (local and systemic). Local complications are mainly pancreatic pseudocyst, acute necrotic collection, acute peripancreatic fluid collection, and walled-off necrosis; systemic complications are defined as multi-organ failure or as an exacerbation of a pre-existing condition [18]. A mean of 15–20% of AP patients will course a severe form of the disease, but mortality is present in only 2–3% of patients because of complications [19, 20].

2. Nutritional support in clinical AP

2.1 Overview

Nutritional therapy and nutritional supplements have great advantages in maintaining the integrity of intestinal barrier, providing major immunomodulatory and antioxidant effects, but more importantly restoring energy balance [21]. The main benefit of nutritional support lies in its immunologic effect, including maintenance of normal intestinal mobility and IgA production, prevention of bacterial overgrowth and infection, diminished bacterial translocation, promoting adequate intestinal permeability [22], decreasing the inflammatory response [22–24], and disease severity, and also promoting a better resolution of the disease process (i.e., duration of systemic inflammation, hospital length of stay) [23, 25]. Clinical evidence suggests that dietary antioxidants and supplements have the potential in protecting against the augmented inflammatory response of the pancreas and oxidative stress during the initial phase of AP. This includes the use of glutamine, antioxidants, probiotics, omega-3 fatty acids, as well as different formulations of enteral and parenteral nutrition [21, 26–28].

2.2 Metabolic response to acute pancreatitis

2.2.1 Inflammation

Nutritional status during AP is affected by several factors, more importantly in the inflammation cascade. It is fed with increased secretion of tumor necrosis factor (TNF) secondary to hypotension, ischemia, endotoxin, hypoxemia, and reperfusion. Nitric oxide synthesis also increased activating the arachidonic acid pathway and inducing the activation of cyclooxygenase (COX). TNF and interleukin (IL) 1 are synergistic, leading to augmented neutrophil activation and permeability [29]. IL-1 also increases T-cell and macrophage activation, fever, and COX and nitric oxide synthase production [29]. IL-8 is an endogenous chemoattractant, present for a longer period, and is notably proinflammatory. IL-6 is frequently used as a biomarker of severity of the inflammatory response. It has both proinflammatory and anti-inflammatory activities [29]. However, the intestinal epithelial barrier is the first line of defense during AP and carries out the production of immunoglobulin A (IgA). Ap is also characterized by causing weakening of this defense system because of increased capillary leakage and decreased activity of tight junctions in preserving the integrity of intestinal barrier secondary to inflammatory mediators. When the intestinal barrier is compromised, intestinal bacteria can penetrate the bloodstream. Invading microorganisms are recognized in minutes by multiple components of innate immunity [29]. Peak inflammatory cytokine production is observed 24–36 hours after initial symptoms of pain, and subsequent systemic manifestations and distant organ failure 2–4 days later [30]. This dysregulation of the immune system leads to a major organic and systemic inflammation and immune paralysis, causing a worsening clinical course during AP [29].

2.2.2 Metabolic changes

Inflammatory cytokines (TNF, IL 1, and 6) as well as stress hormones (cortisol, catecholamines, and glucagon) are produced during AP. As a result, a dysregulation of basal metabolism is similar to trauma or sepsis [23, 31, 32]. When overwhelming inflammation is observed, it produces augmented protein catabolism, characterized by a decremented production of gluconeogenesis by exogenous glucose, increased energy expenditure and insulin resistance, and an augmented dependence of fatty acid oxidation for energy substrates. Energy needs are in constant change according to the severity and stage of AP, comorbidities, as well as complications during the clinical course of AP [23, 32]. In the same sentence, impaired nutrient digestion and absorption occurred during AP produce nutritional deficiencies. This can be particularly severe in undernourished patients, as well as alcoholic patients, who are at great risk of AP. Without the correct and opportune nutritional support, patients develop malnutrition in a rapid manner, as well as water retention and decreased muscle function [33].

In patients with AP, resting energy expenditure (REE) measured by indirect calorimetry (IC) is increased by 61% and by 82% in complicated by infection ± SD of measured REE was 111% ± 15% in mild pancreatitis, 126% ± 10% in SAP, and 120% ± 11% in pancreatic sepsis, compared with predicted REE by Harris-Benedict equation [3]. The substrates for the production of acute-phase occurred during AP covered by amino acid released from protein breakdown observed in about 80% of patients with severe necrotizing pancreatitis [31]. In the same way, nitrogen loss can be up to 20–40 g/d and these patients have a tenfold higher death rate than those with normal balance [34]. Regarding carbohydrate metabolism, hyperglycemia is frequently observed in patients with AP, as a result of an imbalance of insulin resistance, increased hepatic glucose production, and impaired insulin secretion caused by beta-cell damage [35]. Hyperglycemia is associated with necrosis and its infectious complications. Clinical therapy should include blood glucose control in a strict manner [36]. Hypertriglyceridemia is also common during AP, and it can be caused by any complication related to AP, or it can produce pancreatitis. Elevated serum triglycerides and impaired lipid clearance are caused by lipid catabolism, resulting from decreased insulin secretion [36]. Severe hypertriglyceridemia is considered when serum triglycerides > 11.3 mmol/L, and in the absence of gallstones and significant alcohol consumption, it can cause AP [9, 36].

Micronutrient deficiencies are commonly observed in AP. On the other hand, chronic alcohol consumption can cause micronutrient deficiencies due to impaired storage and utilization of nutrients, inadequate intake, and decreased absorption. These deficiencies include vitamin B1, B2, B3, B12, C, A, folic acid, and zinc [37, 38]. Moreover, deficiencies in patients with severe complicated pancreatitis often require hospital admission.

3. Nutritional support in AP

3.1 Nutritional requirements

Energy requirements should be estimated with IC if possible or should be given 25–35 kcal/kg/d as energy goal, the estimated protein requirements range over 1.2–1.5 g/kg/d. This may improve nitrogen balance and is related to a decrease in 28-d mortality in critically ill patients [39]. A mixed source of energy from carbohydrates, fat, and protein should be provided [40, 41]. In severe AP, carbohydrates/day should be 3–6 g/kg and up to 2 g/kg of lipid/day.

3.2 Enteral nutrition vs. parenteral nutrition

Enteral nutrition (EN) is feasible, safe, and beneficial in all types of pancreatitis [42]. It is currently acknowledged that EN properly applied may be essential to enhance AP-associated malnutrition and its general effects; on the other hand, bowel rest has been associated with atrophy of the intestinal mucosa and an increase in infectious complications [43]. About 60% of patients with AP have experienced gut barrier dysfunction [8, 44]. It is important to mention that EN has immunomodulatory effects that preserve the integrity of the intestinal mucosa, in addition to stimulating intestinal motility and reducing the excessive growth of bacteria, [8, 45] and diminishing endotoxin and bacterial translocation [46–49].

The 2016 American Society for Parenteral and Enteral Nutrition/society of critical care medicine guidelines recommend EN over parenteral nutrition (PN) and show a decrease in infectious morbidity (42.6% vs. 16.1%, $P < .0001$) and mortality (16.4% vs. 6.1%, $P = .02$); [50] EN also decreases levels of TNF, IL-1, IL-6, and IL-8 [47]. A meta-analysis of eight randomized clinical trials found that EN considerably reduced mortality, organ failure, and surgical intervention compared with PN [51]. EN vs. PN mortality rates showed an increase in survival with EN (4% vs. 15.9%). In patients with SAP, EN is preferred to PN, whether administered orally or by tube, it preserves the intestinal barrier function to prevent bacterial translocation. The New England Journal of Medicine demonstrated, in a multicenter randomized study, that both early tube feeding and oral diet after 72 hours given to patients with AP at high risk of complications are equivalent in reducing infection rates or death [46]. Multiple meta-analyses have been found that support the use of EN in PN, such as a Cochrane study in which eight randomized controlled studies were carried out in patients with PA comparing EN with PN, it was found that EN reduced mortality, systemic infections, and multi-organ failure [52]. Another study carried out on 381 patients confirmed the benefit of EN over PN in patients with SAP, and the results showed lower mortality, fewer infectious complications, a lower rate of organ failure, and surgical intervention [49]. Several trials have suggested that the optimal EN route is the nasogastric route, putting it as an alternative to the nasoduodenal or nasojejunal routes [53–55]. As demonstrated in multiple trials involving a sample of 157 SAP patients, the results were that nasogastric feeding is safe and well tolerated compared with nasojejunal feeding [41, 56]. Nevertheless, as shown by multiple randomized trials that have associated total PN (TPN) with risks of infection and other complications [57]. PN should still be minimized unless the enteral route is not available, not tolerated, or not meeting caloric requirements [58, 59]. PN causes increased inflammatory cytokines, leading to a proinflammatory state in the gastrointestinal tract [58, 60]. Overall, PN is more expensive than EN or oral nutrition and associated with more complications [61].

3.3 Nutrition support in mild and moderate AP

In the care of patients with mild-to-moderate AP, food can be given orally once nausea, vomiting, and abdominal pain have subsided and appetite has returned [62, 63]. The conventional way of feeding patients with AP is increasing, that is, once the abdominal pain has disappeared and the pancreatic enzymes have decreased, the first 24 hours are given clear liquids to later consume a low-fat soft diet for 24 hours to check tolerance, and then start a solid low-fat diet [57]. However, a randomized study determined that providing a soft diet with clear liquids to patients with mild AP did not show significant differences in the two participating groups. In addition, it was determined that starting treatment with a solid diet is associated with a shorter hospital stay (mean of 5 vs. 8 days of starting with clear liquids, $p < 0.001$) . On the other hand, a current open-label randomized trial [64] demonstrated no difference in tolerance to refeeding when comparing both the stepped and immediate full-calorie diets. Likewise, it was mentioned that fasting caused by constant abdominal pain in patients with moderate AP should not exceed five days, and if this is the case, a catheter should be placed [62, 63, 65].

Theory mentions that nasojejunal feeding is preferred over nasogastric feeding because it is assumed to be more tolerable for patients [66]. In nasojejunal feeding, placing the tube in the jejunum beyond the duodenum avoids stimulation of the already inflamed pancreas, causing less pain. However, there are studies that compared nasojejunal and nasogastric feeding and did not find significant differences [67, 68]. The current indication is that continuous feeding over bolus feeding is recommended for patients requiring tube feeding [3, 66]. EN demonstrated better feeding tolerance and decreased interruptions due to high residuals and vomiting in the continuous infusion when compared with the bolus group [69, 70].

The method of administration of the nasogastric diet is through interrupted boluses (200–300 mL 5–6 times a day) under control of gastric residual volume (GRV) or continuous infusion (30–50 mL/h), unlike NE via NJT that is administered in continuous infusions. Gradually increasing the flow rate: from 20 to 30 ml/h to 100 to 125 ml/h. To avoid complications (regurgitation, aspiration, or pneumonia), EN *via* the nasogastric route should be interrupted at GRV > 200 mL. The EN must cover a minimum of 60% of the energy requirement. When intolerance to EN occurs, resulting in effects such as diarrhea, the rate of feed delivery should be decreased. When this is not enough, a switch to EN should be considered. The continuous evaluation of the nutritional requirement and the laboratory investigations must be carried out weekly with the objective of optimally carrying out the nutritional support and if required, the modification of the type or formula if indicated. In addition, it is essential to carry out adequate care of the tube (in EN) or catheter (in PN) to avoid infections and other complications related to the catheter and the tube [1, 71]. Due to its nature, parenteral nutrition is reserved only for patients who present intolerance or are unable to receive enteral nutrition [52, 72].

3.4 Nutrition support in severe AP

At the international level [62, 63, 65, 73, 74], it is mentioned that in patients with SAP, nutritional support should be provided through enteral feeding (grade of recommendation: A). Even if complications such as fistulas, ascites, and pseudocysts occur, EN is preferred over PN (grade of recommendation: C) [63, 65]. After surgery for pancreatitis, EN is recommended through intraoperative jejunostomy (grade of recommendation: C) [65]. Since enteral tube feeding can provide safe nutritional support in AP even in cases where gastric outlet is obstructed [75] in this case, the tip of the tube should be placed distal to the obstruction (grade of recommendation: C) [65]. However, early EN (enteral tube feeding within 24 hours of presentation) has not been shown to improve outcomes in SAP patients, compared with oral feeding starting at 72 hours. [76]

The only real contraindication to EN is prolonged paralytic ileus. However, according to the European Society for Parenteral and Enteral Nutrition guidelines, it is advisable to combine PN with a small content of an elemental or immunopotentiating diet (10–30 ml/h) continuously infused into the jejunum. Regarding delivery times, continuous infusion is preferred over bolus administration (grade B recommendation) [65, 66].

3.5 Time of enteral support

EN should be initiated when the patient has an established condition for gut permeability and should start after adequate resuscitation and stable hemodynamic status. Many studies have shown the advantages of early enteral feeding in SAP and how convenient it is for the prognosis [77]. A meta-analysis conducted by Petrov [78] showed that the timely administration of EN during the first 48 hours of admission improved the reduction of multiorgan failure, complications of infectious origin, and mortality rate in comparison with PN. After this period, there were no significant differences observed in comparison with PN. Starting EN before 48 hours provide several advantages in more successive studies and another meta-analysis. Many studies have shown this association, and a more recent meta-analysis, improving the time, demonstrated that starting EN within 24 hours after hospital admission was associated with lower complications for predicted severe or SAP, but not for mild to moderate pancreatitis. [76, 79–82]. A multicenter randomized controlled trial compared early EN within 24 h versus an on-demand oral diet of 72 h, with tube feeding provided on day 4 if the oral diet was not tolerated. This study showed that patients with moderate pancreatitis, who do not require intensive care, can use an oral diet on demand and only through a tube from day 4 if the oral diet is not successful [76].

3.6 Gastric vs. small bowel feeding

In response to decreased efficiency in pancreatic secretion during PA, nasogastric feeding has been considered to be similar to nasojejunal feeding when the following parameters are assessed: pain, aspiration, compliance with energy balance, and mortality; this even though it was previously believed that feeding through the small intestine could decrease the stimulation of the pancreas and digestion [55].

Feeding in the stomach is the most used because it is easier and cheaper, and it optimizes the time for the patient who requires EN, since through the intestine, not only a special technique is required, but also more time for the correct one tube placement. However, this technique is mainly used for patients who do not tolerate gastric feedings, such as obstructions, edema, severe gastroparesis, or pseudocysts. Likewise, the use of jejunal probes is indicated for post-operative patients in different conditions where it is required [65, 83].

3.7 Polymeric vs. semielemental formula

Formulations used in EN and PN are compounds based on the following nutritional requirements: protein 1.2–1.5 g/kg/d, carbohydrates 3–6 g/kg/d (glucose concentration, aim: <10 mmol/L), lipids up to 2 g/kg/day, (triglyceride concentration, aim: <12 mmol/L), Natrium 1–2 mmol/kg/d, potassium 1–2 mmol/kg/d, chlorine 2–4 mmol/kg/d, phosphorus 0.1–0.5 mmol/kg/d, magnesium 0.1–0.2 mmol/kg/d, and calcium 0.1 mmol/kg/d. Naturally, this formula could be adapted for the clinical condition of the patient, depending on the above-mentioned serum concentrations [79]. Enteral formulas are classified into elemental (monomeric), semi-elemental (oligomeric), and standard (polymeric) formulas and differ in protein and fat concentration. Elemental formulas contain amino acids, simple sugars, and very low fats; semi-elemental formulas contain peptides of various chain lengths, a simple sugar, glucose polymers or starch, and medium-chain triglycerides, and polymeric formulas contain intact proteins, complex carbohydrates, and long-chain triglycerides [84].

Nevertheless, polymeric formulas are safe and comply with the same nutrimental function as elemental and semi-elemental formulas if administered *via* nasojejunal tube in AP patients [85–87]. A meta-analysis by Petrov et al including 1070 patients found no significant difference in feeding tolerance (RR = 0.62; 95%CI: 0.10–3.97), infection (RR = 0.48; 95%CI: 0.06–3.76), and death (RR = 0.63; 95%CI: 0.04–9.86) [85–89]. It should be remembered that semi-elemental or elemental formulas are at least sevenfold as expensive as polymeric feeds [90, 77, 91].

3.8 Parenteral nutrition

EN is the first way of nutrition, however, if it is not possible to use it or there is intolerance to it, parental nutrition (PN) can be used, which is used after the fifth or seventh day of admission to increasing, in this way, the correct clinical development of the patient and decrease the hospitalization days [40, 59, 89, 92, 93] EN intolerance is generally accompanied by diarrhea and in such cases, PN nutrition is considered. It is recommended that PN must have a gradual increment starting from day one up to day three in the following way 50%, 75%, and 100%, and must include carbohydrates, proteins, and lipids. The control of the hemodynamic status of the patients has to be overseen even before starting the nutrition in order to avoid the re-feeding syndrome in such a way that the formula can be readapted if required [1].

An important consideration is that glucose should not be more than the maximal level of glucose oxidation (4–7 mg/kg/min or 5–6 g/kg/d), and a target blood glucose range of 7.7–10 mmol/L is recommended [94, 95]. Intravenous lipid emulsions can be safely started, and the recommended dose is 0.8–1.5 g/kg/d [40, 41]. Intravenous lipid emulsions dose may need to be reduced or discontinued if serum triglyceride consent iterations are greater than 4.5 mmol/L [96, 97]. In PN-exclusive nutrition, a daily dose of multivitamins and trace elements should be administered. Micronutrients should be supplemented in patients with confirmed or suspected deficiencies of estimated nutritional requirements gradually from day 1 to day 3. The hemodynamic status must be watched to avoid water/electrolyte and acid-base imbalances [1, 41].

4. Nutritional supplements and antioxidants in AP

Various supplements such as probiotics, glutamine, omega-3 fatty acids, and different formulations of enteral and parenteral nutrition have been studied with the aim of reducing inflammation and improving outcomes in AP [28]; however, their clinical benefit is still unclear.

4.1 Vitamins

AP carries great oxidative stress and an acute systemic inflammatory response, [98] which is the reason why it is suggested that patients with AP have lower serum levels of anti-oxidant vitamins and may benefit from supplementation [99]. Vitamin A, vitamin C, vitamin E, selenium, and N-acetyl cysteine are important immunonutrients and have been inversely associated with AP [98]. It has been described that they may reduce inflammation and improve outcomes in SAP. Nevertheless, only a few small studies with varied doses and duration of vitamins have studied this effect with non-conclusive results: Musil et al. [21] found that plasma concentrations of vitamin A and vitamin C were significantly lower in AP patients compared with controls ($P < 0.05$) [100]. Recently, another study reported that vitamin D has been inversely associated with gallstone-related AP [98].

It has also been assessed the vitamin supplementation in combination with other antioxidants or in vitamin-only therapy and yielded mixed outcomes: In a multicenter randomized, double-blind, placebo clinical trial by Siriwardena et al. the use of intravenous combination of antioxidant therapy containing vitamin C, was not clinically justified to continue in AP [101]. Subsequently, another group comparing vitamin C (N-acetylcysteine) in combination with standard medical treatment in early AP suggested that antioxidant supplementation reduced the length of hospital stay and complications in these patients [102].

Another study with high vitamin C doses, involving 84 AP patients and 40 healthy subjects in China, demonstrated therapeutic efficacy on the disease, and they proposed that promoting anti-oxidizing capability in these patients, may block lipid peroxidation and improve cellular immune function [103]. This hypothesis cannot yet be proven, as another group studied multiple vitamin-based antioxidant therapy (vitamin A, vitamin C, and vitamin E) in a randomized study involving 39 patients, in which there was no proven benefit [104].

4.2 Curcumin

Curcumin (CUR) has been described as an important antioxidant, anti-apoptotic, anti-cancer, and anti-inflammatory supplement, [105–109], acting as a free radical scavenger [42, 110], and increases the expression of anti-oxidant enzymes like superoxide dismutase (SOD), catalase (CAT), glutathione peroxidase (GPx), hemo oxygenase-1 (HO-1), and others [111]. Also, CUR exerts an anti-inflammatory effect through its ability to diminish the activation of nuclear factor κ B (NFκB, p65/p50), [112], which reduces the expression of inflammatory cytokines like IL-1β, IL-6, TNFα, cyclo-oxygenase 2, lipoxygenase 5, and inducible nitric oxide synthase [113].

In experimental models of AP, CUR decreased the level of serum amylase, the number of myeloperoxidase, NFκB, and apoptotic cells. Furthermore, pancreatic inflammation, edema, and necrosis of fat cells also decreased after inducing pancreatitis with L-arginine. Histopathological features in experimental pancreatitis were normalized by effect of CUR [114]. Similar findings were reported by Yu [115] in an AP induced with caerulein. Finally, a clinical study in tropical pancreatitis suggested the beneficial effect of CUR by decreasing the level of lipid peroxidation and reinforcing the activation of the endogenous antioxidant enzymes [116]. Thus, the potential benefits of CUR alone or combined with other antioxidants contained in micro or nano-formulations [116] continue to be evaluated and applied in AP.

4.3 Gut microbiome impact in AP

The human gastrointestinal tract has a rich microbiota, consisting of a vast number of microorganisms and >5000 genes. About 80–90% of the gut microbiome are Firmicutes and Bacteroidetes, being the most prevalent bacteria [55]. The gut microbiome influences the immune system through its effect on systemic metabolism.

In acute pancreatitis, the microbiome is altered by the increased intestinal permeability [117], resulting in important dysbiosis [118]. Changes in the intestinal microbiota during AP depend on the course of the disease, with a decrease in the diversity of microorganisms in acute necrotic pancreatitis [119]. Also, the need for aggressive medical therapy with acid suppression and reduced oral feeding creates a microbial imbalance [117, 118].

Increased intestinal permeability has been demonstrated in a significant percentage of patients with AP [120], with circulating bacterial DNA representative of gut bacteria in 68.8% of patients with AP. Zhang and colleagues showed that patients with AP had more Proteobacteria and Bacteroidetes and fewer Actinobacteria and Firmicutes in their feces, compared with normal controls [121]. The clinical significance of gut dysbiosis is poorly understood, but these patients have been found to have worse outcomes .

Mechanisms of microbiome alteration include 1. poor intestinal mobility: resulting in the growth of Gram negative and anaerobic microflora, in addition to the accumulation of substances that will inhibit the growth of probiotics, [122]. 2. Gut mucosal ischemia: Inflammation in the environment generated by AP can cause ischemia injury due to the release of proinflammatory cytokines, which together, with the increased migration of cells of the immune system, alters the microbiota destroying the bacterial glycocalyx [123]. 3. Oxidative stress: The subsequent inflammation in the tissue leads to the release of reactive oxygen species, and the oxidative state present in the tissue allows the presence of oxygen-tolerant bacteria [124].

Different strategies are recommended to recover the intestinal microbiome in the treatment of AP, mainly with the use of probiotics. These are live microorganisms that confer a health benefit through the inhibition of pathogenic microorganisms, the induction of growth of the mucous layer, and inhibiting apoptosis of epithelial cells. The most used probiotics are Lactobacillus, Bifidobacterium, Streptococcus, and Lactococcus lactis among others [125, 126]. Other strategies as antibiotics are not widely used in patients with AP since their prophylactic use does not reduce mortality, and in spite of this, Ahuja et al. [127] reported that the pancreatic acini were able to regulate the intestinal microbiota through the secretion of antimicrobials and different pro-inflammatory cytokines, which still must be proven.

4.4 Glutamine

For unfed sterocytes, glutamine represents an important substrate [30]. Long-term parenteral nutrition can cause glutamine deficiency, which in turn leads to intestinal dysfunction [47]. Supplementing PN with glutamine is recommended for patients with critical illnesses associated with a catabolic response, as it helps preserve the cell mass of the stomach-associated lymphatic tissue and antibacterial defenses [30, 51].

It has been shown that glutamine can be associated with a decrease in infectious complications, as a result of a meta-analysis of 12 RCTs (RR = 0.58; 95% CI: 0.39–0.87) and mortality (RR = 0 .30, 95% CI: 0.15–0.60). In this study, statistically significant benefits were shown among patients who received total PN but not EN [128]. The above findings were confirmed in another study that determined the advantages of intravenous glutamine [129]. Among the most recent studies was found that enteral glutamine showed an improvement in the organ failure score, it did not obtain significant benefits in infected necrosis and mortality [130]. One study showed that giving PN with glutamine supplementation reduced overall complications by 25% compared to the PN-only group by 47% [131]. Overall, giving intravenous glutamine appears to be beneficial in patients with total PN, however, the beneficial effects of enteral glutamine should be investigated in the future. Glutamine is recommended as a supplement in the following doses 0.3 to 0.5 g/kg/d [130, 132, 133].

4.5 Omega-3 fatty acids

Remarkable immunomodulatory benefits are described from dietary polyunsaturated fatty acids, especially lipoxins, resolvins, and protectins, [134, 135]

A randomized study found that enteral formula enriched with ω-3 FA in the treatment of AP reduced the total time of jejunal feeding and hospital length [136]. Also, more studies evaluated the effects of ω-3 FA supplemented in the PN during SAP. Wang et al. performed a randomized, double-blind trial of 40 SAP patients receiving PN with the same amount of nutrients but different lipid contents, including soybean oil-/fish oil-based fat solutions. It was observed that patients with ω-3 FAs-supplemented PN had higher levels of eicosapentaenoic acid and decreased pro-inflammatory cytokines, together with improved respiratory function and a minor renal replacement therapy time, suggesting an attenuated systemic response to pancreatic and organ injury [137]. Another study by the same authors who included 56 patients receiving an isocaloric and isonitrogenous PN with fats of all ω-6 FAs or

4:1 ω-6:ω-3 FAs demonstrated that ω-3 FAs-supplemented PN augmented the expression of IL-10, and human leukocyte antigen-DR in SAP patients [137]. In the same way, during the first hours of SAP, supplementation with ω-3 fish oil emulsion in PN decreased SIRS, and improved the balance of pro-/anti-inflammatory cytokines and thus improved AP-associated severe [138]. Moreover, a meta-analysis of eight small RCTs showed that omega-3 fatty acids supplementation was beneficial in the total mortality, infectious complications, and length of hospital stay, especially when received parenterally. Nonetheless, large and well-designed RCTs are required to elucidate the efficacy of omega-3 FA supplementation during SAP.

5. Conclusions

Nutritional therapy since the onset of AP constitutes a critical component in the management of patients that should be performed and assessed in the first hours of hospital admission. If the patient has mild disease and the on-demand oral diet of low-fat solid foods is tolerated, and not limited to clear liquids or if the enteral nutrition support is well tolerated during SAP, a daily reassessment of tolerance should be performed. The correct time to start enteral support should be performed in the first 24–48 hours after onset of AP. In contrast, early EN may not be better than an on-demand oral diet at 72 h. If it is not tolerated, then the enteral route through a nasogastric or nasojejunal feeding tube should be attempted. The use of a standard polymeric formula is recommended in gastric and jejunal feeding; nonetheless, daily assessment of tolerance should be carried out. PN is considered the last option because of the considerable risks of infection, and other complications. Lastly, various nutritional supplements used during AP have mixed clinical outcomes that should be more elucidated to bring certainty of their use to achieve better clinical outcomes.

Conflict of interest

The authors declare no conflict of interest.

Acronyms and abbreviations

AP	acute pancreatitis
SAP	severe acute pancreatitis
TNF	tumor necrosis factor
COX	cyclooxygenase
IL	interleukin
REE	resting energy expenditure
IC	indirect calorimetry
EN	enteral nutrition
PN	parenteral nutrition
TPN	total parenteral nutrition
GRV	gastric residual volume

Author details

Mariana Chávez-Tostado[1*], Karla Verónica Chávez-Tostado[2], Clotilde Fuentes-Orozco[3], Alejandro González-Ojeda[3], María Luisa Mendoza-Magaña[4], Mario Alberto Ramírez-Herrera[4], Gabino Cervantes-Guevara[5], Guillermo Alonso Cervantes-Cardona[6], Enrique Cervantes-Pérez[7], Diana Mercedes Hernández-Corona[8], Tonatiuh González-Heredia[8], Miriam Méndez-del Villar[8], María Fernanda Isadora Meraz-Corona[8], Milton Omar Guzmán-Ornelas[8], Abraham Alberto Ramírez-Mendoza[4] and Steffany Arandeni Ramírez-Mendoza[4]

1 Departamento de Clínicas de la Reproducción Humana, Crecimiento y Desarrollo Infantil, Centro Universitario de Ciencias de la Salud, Universidad de Guadalajara, Guadalajara, México

2 Departamento de Cirugía, Hospital Regional "Lic. Adolfo López Mateos," México

3 Unidad de Investigación Biomédica 02, Hospital de Especialidades, Centro Médico Nacional de Occidente, Instituto Mexicano del Seguro Social, Guadalajara, México

4 Departamento de Fisiología, Laboratorio de Neurofisiología, Centro Universitario de Ciencias de la Salud, Universidad de Guadalajara, Guadalajara, México

5 Departamento de Gastroenterología, Hospital Civil de Guadalajara "Fray Antonio Alcalde", Guadalajara, México

6 Departamento de Disciplinas Filosóficas, Metodológicas e Instrumentales, Centro Universitario de Ciencias de la Salud, Universidad de Guadalajara, Guadalajara, México

7 Departamento de Medicina Interna, Hospital Civil de Guadalajara "Fray Antonio Alcalde", Guadalajara, México

8 Departamento de Ciencias Biomédicas, Centro de Investigación Multidisciplinario en Salud, Centro Universitario de Tonalá, Universidad de Guadalajara, Tonalá, México

*Address all correspondence to: ln.marianachavez@gmail.com

References

[1] Jabłońska B, Mrowiec S. Nutritional support in patients with severe acute pancreatitis-current standards. Nutrients. 2021;**13**(5):1498

[2] McClave SA, Snider H, Owens N, Sexton LK. Clinical nutrition in pancreatitis. Digestive Diseases and Sciences. 1997;**42**(10):2035-2044

[3] Dickerson RN, Vehe KL, Mullen JL, Feurer ID. Resting energy expenditure in patients with pancreatitis. Critical Care Medicine. 1991;**19**(4):484-490

[4] Abou-Assi S, O'Keefe SJ. Nutrition support during acute pancreatitis. Nutrition. 2002;**18**(11-12):938-943

[5] Abou-Assi S, O'Keefe SJ. Nutrition in acute pancreatitis. Journal of Clinical Gastroenterology. 2001;**32**(3):203-209

[6] Lodewijkx PJ, Besselink MG, Witteman BJ, Schepers NJ, Gooszen HG, van Santvoort HC. Nutrition in acute pancreatitis: A critical review. Expert Review of Gastroenterology & Hepatology. 2016;**10**(5):571-580

[7] Yadav D, Lowenfels AB. The epidemiology of pancreatitis and pancreatic cancer. Gastroenterology. Gastroenterology. 2013;**144**:1252-1261

[8] Lankisch PG, Apte M, Banks PA. Acute pancreatitis. Lancet. 2015;**386**:85-96. DOI: 10.1016/S0140-6736(14)60649-8

[9] Tenner S, Baillie J, DeWitt J, Vege SS, American College of Gastroenterology. American College of Gastroenterology guideline: Management of acute pancreatitis. The American Journal of Gastroenterology. 2013;**108**:1400-1415

[10] Gravante G, Garcea G, Ong SL, Metcalfe MS, Berry DP, Lloyd DM, et al. Prediction of mortality in acute pancreatitis: A systematic review of the published evidence. Pancreatology. 2009;**9**:601-614. DOI: 10.1159/000212097

[11] van Santvoort HC, Bakker OJ, Bollen TL, et al. A conservative and minimally invasive approach to necrotizing pancreatitis improves outcome. Gastroenterology. 2011;**141**(4):1254-1263

[12] Petrov MS, Shanbhag S, Chakraborty M, Phillips AR, Windsor JA. Organ failure and infection of pancreatic necrosis as determinants of mortality in patients with acute pancreatitis. Gastroenterology. 2010;**139**(3):813-820

[13] Zuo YY, Kang Y, Yin WH, Wang B, Chen Y. The association of mean glucose level and glucose variability with intensive care unit mortality in patients with severe acute pancreatitis. Journal of Critical Care. 2012;**27**(2):146-152

[14] Vujasinovic M, Tepes B, Makuc J, et al. Pancreatic exocrine insufficiency, diabetes mellitus and serum nutritional markers after acute pancreatitis. World Journal of Gastroenterology: WJG. 2014;**20**(48):18432-18438

[15] da Costa DW, Boerma D, van Santvoort HC, et al. Staged multidisciplinary step-up management for necrotizing pancreatitis. The British Journal of Surgery. 2014;**101**(1):e65-e79

[16] Banks PA, Bollen TL, Dervenis C, Gooszen HG, Johnson CD, Sarr MG, et al. Classification of acute pancreatitis–2012: Revision of the Atlanta classification and definitions by international consensus. Gut. 2013;**62**:102-111

[17] Lee PJ, Papachristou GI. New insights into acute pancreatitis. Nature Reviews. Gastroenterology & Hepatology. 2019 Aug;**16**(8):479-496

[18] Forsmark CE, Baillie J. AGA institute technical review on acute pancreatitis. Gastroenterology. 2007;**132**:2022-2044

[19] Russo MW, Wei JT, Thiny MT, Gangarosa LM, Brown A, Ringel Y, et al. Digestive and liver diseases statistics, 2004. Gastroenterology. 2004; **126**:1448-1453

[20] Woodcock S, Siriwardena A. High early mortality rate from acute pancreatitis in Scotland, 1984-95. The British Journal of Surgery. 2000;**87**:379-380

[21] Pan LL, Li J, Shamoon M, Bhatia M, Sun J. Recent advances on nutrition in treatment of acute pancreatitis. Frontiers in Immunology. 2017;**8**:762

[22] van Dijk SM, Hallensleben NDL, van Santvoort HC, et al. Acute pancreatitis: Recent advances through randomised trials. Gut. 2017;**66**(11):2024-2032

[23] Murphy AE, Codner PA. Acute pancreatitis: Exploring nutrition implications. Nutrition in Clinical Practice. 2020;**35**(5):807-817

[24] Li XY, He C, Zhu Y, Lu NH. Role of gut microbiota on intestinal barrier function in acute pancreatitis. World Journal of Gastroenterology. 2020;**26**(18):2187-2193

[25] Hegazi RA, DeWitt T. Enteral nutrition and immune modulation of acute pancreatitis. World Journal of Gastroenterology. 2014;**20**(43):16101-16105

[26] McClave SA, Chang WK, Dhaliwal R, et al. Nutrition support in acute pancreatitis: A systematic review of the literature. JPEN Journal of Parenteral and Enteral Nutrition. 2006;**30**(2):143-156

[27] Youdim KA, Joseh JA. A possible emerging role of phytochemicals in improving age-related neurological dysfunctions: A multiplicity of effects. Free Radical Biology & Medicine. 2001;**30**(6):583-594

[28] McClave SA, Heyland DK. The physiologic response and associated clinical benefits from provision of early enteral nutrition. Nutrition in Clinical Practice. 2009;**24**(3):305-315

[29] Lenz A, Franklin GA, Cheadle WG. Systemic inflammation after trauma. Injury. 2007;**38**(12):1336-1345

[30] Barash M, Jayshil JP. Gut luminal and clinical benefits of early enteral nutrition in shock. Current Surgery Report. 2019;**7**(10):21

[31] Shaw JH, Wolfe RR. Glucose, fatty acid, and urea kinetics in patients with severe pancreatitis. The response to substrate infusion and total parenteral nutrition. Annals of Surgery. 1986;**204**:665-672

[32] Fuchs-Tarlovsky V, Sriram K. Nutrition Assessment and Therapy in Acute Pancreatitis. In: Rodrigo L, editor. Acute Pancreatitis [Internet]. London: IntechOpen; 2012 [cited 2022 Aug 29]. Available from: https://www.intechopen.com/chapters/26195 doi: 10.5772/26577

[33] Rinninella E, Annetta MG, Serricchio ML, Dal Lago AA, Miggiano GA, Mele MC. Nutritional support in acute pancreatitis: From physiopathology to practice. An evidence-based approach. European Review for Medical and Pharmacological Sciences. 2017;**21**(2):421-432

[34] Sitzmann JV, Steinborn PA, Zinner MJ, Cameron JL. Total parenteral nutrition and alternate energy substrates in treatment of severe acute pancreatitis. Surgery, Gynecology & Obstetrics. 1989;**168**:311-317

[35] Solomon SS, Duckworth WC, Jallepalli P, Bobal MA, Iyer R. The glucose intolerance of acute pancreatitis: Hormonal response to arginine. Diabetes. 1980;**29**:22-26

[36] Meier RF, Beglinger C. Nutrition in pancreatic diseases. Best Practice & Research. Clinical Gastroenterology. 2006;**20**:507-529

[37] Lugli AK, Carli F, Wykes L. The importance of nutrition status assessment: The case of severe acute pancreatitis. Nutrition Reviews. 2007;**65**:329-334

[38] De Waele B, Vierendeels T, Willems G. Vitamin status in patients with acute pancreatitis. Clinical Nutrition. 1992;**11**:83-86

[39] Allingstrup MJ, Esmailzadeh N, Wilkens Knudsen A, Espersen K, Hartvig Jensen T, Wiis J, et al. Provision of protein and energy in relation to measured requirements in intensive care patients. Clinical Nutrition. 2012;**31**:462-468

[40] Krueger K, McClave SA, Martindale RG. Pancreatitis. In: Mueller CM, editor. The ASPEN Adult Nutrition Support Core Curriculum. 3rd ed. United States: American Society for Parenteral and Enteral Nutrition; 2017. pp. 549-564

[41] Gianotti L, Meier R, Lobo DN, Bassi C, Dejong CH, Ockenga J, et al. ESPEN guidelines on parenteral nutrition: Pancreas. Clinical Nutrition. 2009;**28**:428-435

[42] Priyadarsini KI. The chemistry of curcumin: From extraction to therapeutic agent. Molecules. 2014;**19**:20091

[43] Peery AF, Crockett SD, Barritt AS, Dellon ES, Eluri S, Gangarosa LM, et al. Burden of gastrointestinal, liver, and pancreatic diseases in the United States. Gastroenterology. 2015;**149**:1731

[44] Sendler M et al. Cathepsin B-mediated activation of trypsinogen in endocytosing macrophages increases severity of pancreatitis in mice. Gastroenterology. 2018;**154**:704-718

[45] Zeng Y, Wang X, Zhang W, Wu K, Ma J. Hypertriglyceridemia aggravates ER stress and pathogenesis of acute pancreatitis. Hepato-Gastroenterology. 2012;**59**:2318-2326

[46] Márta K, Szabó AN, Pécsi D, et al. High versus low energy administration in the early phase of acute pancreatitis (GOULASH trial): Protocol of a multicentre randomised double-blind clinical trial. BMJ Open. 2017;7(9):e015874

[47] Shen QX, Xu GX, Shen MH. Effect of early enteral nutrition (EN) on endotoxin in serum and intestinal permeability in patients with severe acute pancreatitis. European Review for Medical and Pharmacological Sciences. 2017;**21**(11):2764-2768

[48] Stimac D, Poropat G, Hauser G, et al. Early nasojejunal tube feeding versus nil-by-mouth in acute pancreatitis: A randomized clinical trial. Pancreatology. 2016;**16**(4):523-528

[49] Keefe J, Lee B, Derson P, Gennin C, Bo-Assi S, Clore J, et al. Physiological effects of enteral and parenteral feeding on pancreaticobiliary secretion in humans. American Journal of Physiology. Gastrointestinal and Liver Physiology. 2003;**284**:G27-G36

[50] McClave SA. Drivers of oxidative stress in acute pancreatitis. JPEN Journal of Parenteral and Enteral Nutrition. 2012;**36**(1):24-35

[51] Oláh A, Laszlo R Jr. Enteral nutrition in acute pancreatitis: A review of the current evidence. World Journal of Gastroenterology. 2014;**20**(43):16123

[52] Al-Omran M, Albalawi ZH, Tashkandi MF, Al-Ansary LA. Enteral versus parenteral nutrition for acute pancreatitis. Cochrane Database of Systematic Reviews. 2010;**1**:CD002837

[53] Yi F, Ge L, Zhao J, Lei Y, Zhou F, Chen Z, et al. Meta-analysis: Total parenteral nutrition versus total enteral nutrition in predicted severe acute pancreatitis. Internal Medicine. 2012;**51**:523-530

[54] Wu BU, Banks PA. Clinical management of patients with acute pancreatitis. Gastroenterology. 2013;**144**:1272-1281

[55] Chang YS, Fu HQ, Xiao YM, Liu JC. Nasogastric or nasojejunal feeding in predicted severe acute pancreatitis: A meta-analysis. Critical Care. 2013;**17**:R118

[56] Klek S, Sierzega M, Turczynowski L, et al. Enteral and parenteral nutrition in the conservative treatment of pancreatic fistula: A randomized clinical trial. Gastroenterology. 2011;**141**(1):157-163

[57] Sathiaraj E, Murthy S, Mansard MJ, et al. Clinical trial: Oral feeding with a soft diet compared with clear liquid diet as initial meal in mild acute pancreatitis. Alimentary Pharmacology & Therapeutics. 2008;**28**(6):77781

[58] Madaria E, Herrera-Marante I, González-Camacho V, et al. Fluid resuscitation with lactated Ringer's solution vs normal saline in acute pancreatitis: A triple-blind, randomized, controlled trial. United European Gastroenterology Journal. 2018;**6**:63-72

[59] van Baal MC, van Santvoort HC, Bollen TL, Bakker OJ, Besselink MG, Gooszen HG. Systematic review of percutaneous catheter drainage as primary treatment for necrotizing pancreatitis. The British Journal of Surgery. 2011;**98**:18-27

[60] Besselink MGH, Verwer TJ, Schoenmaeckers EJ, et al. Timing of surgical intervention in necrotizing pancreatitis. Archives of Surgery. 2007;**142**:1194-1201

[61] van Brunschot S, Hollemans RA, Bakker OJ, et al. Minimally invasive and endoscopic versus open necrosectomy for necrotising pancreatitis: A pooled analysis of individual data for 1980 patients. Gut. 2018;**67**:697-706

[62] Greenberg JA, Hsu J, Bawazeer M, Marshall J, Friedrich JO, Nathens A, et al. Clinical practice guideline: Management of acute pancreatitis. Canadian Journal of Surgery. 2016;**59**:128-140

[63] Mirtallo JM, Forbes A, McClave SA, Jensen GL, Waitzberg DL, Davies AR, et al. International consensus guidelines for nutrition therapy in pancreatitis. JPEN Journal of Parenteral and Enteral Nutrition. 2012;**36**:284-291

[64] Lariño-Noia J, Lindkvist B, Iglesias-García J, Seijo-Ríos S, Iglesias-Canle J, Domínguez-Muñoz JE. Early and/ or immediately full caloric diet versus standard refeeding in mild acute pancreatitis: A randomized open-label trial. Pancreatology. 2014;**14**:167-173

[65] Meier R, Ockenga J, Pertkiewicz M, Pap A, Milinic N, Macfie J. ESPEN Guidelines on Enteral Nutrition: Pancreas. Clinical Nutrition. 2006;**25**:275-284

[66] Machicado JD et al. Practice patterns and utilization of tube feedings in acute pancreatitis patients at a large US referral center. Pancreas. 2018;**47**:1150-1155

[67] Eatock FC et al. A randomized study of early nasogastric versus nasojejunal feeding in severe acute pancreatitis. The American Journal of Gastroenterology. 2005;**100**:432-439

[68] Petrov MS, Correia MITD, Windsor JA. Nasogastric tube feeding in predicted severe acute pancreatitis: A systematic review of the literature to determine safety and tolerance. JOP. 2008;**9**:440-448

[69] Steevens EC, Lipscomb AF, Poole GV, Sacks GS. Comparison of continuous vs intermittent nasogastric enteral feeding in trauma patients: Perceptions and practice. Nutrition in Clinical Practice. 2002;**17**:118-122

[70] Van Dyck L, Casaer MP. Intermittent or continuous feeding: Any difference during the first week? Current Opinion in Critical Care. 2019;**25**:356-362

[71] Jab B. Standard akredytacyjny. Zasady Zywienia Dojelitowego I Pozajelitowego. Katowice, Poland: UCK SUM; 2021. pp. 1-16

[72] Yao H, He C, Deng L, Liao G. Enteral versus parenteral nutrition in critically ill patients with severe pancreatitis: A meta-analysis. European Journal of Clinical Nutrition. 2018;**72**:66-68

[73] Meier R, Belin C, Yer P. ESPEN guidelines on nutrition in acute pancreatitis. European Society of Parenteral and Enteral Nutrition. Clinical Nutrition. 2002;**21**:173183

[74] Pezzilli R, Zerbi A, Campra D, Capurso G, Golfieri R, Arcidiacono PG, et al. Consensus guidelines on severe acute pancreatitis. Italian Association for the Study of the Pancreas (AISP). Digestive and Liver Disease. 2015;**47**:532-543

[75] O'Keefe S, Rolniak S, Raina A, Graham T, Hegazi R, Centa-Wagner P. Enteral feeding patients with gastric outlet obstruction. Nutrition in Clinical Practice. 2012;**27**:76-81

[76] Bakker OJ, van Brunschot S, van Santvoort HC, Besselink MG, Bollen TL, Boermeester MA, et al. Early versus on-demand nasoenteric tube feeding in acute pancreatitis. The New England Journal of Medicine. 2014;**371**:1983-1993. DOI: 10.1056/ NEJMoa1404393

[77] Lakananurak N, Gramlich L. Nutrition management in acute pancreatitis: Clinical practice consideration. World Journal of Clinical Cases. 2020;**8**:1561-1573

[78] Petrov MS, Pylypchuk RD, Uchugina AF. A systematic review on the timing of artificial nutrition in acute pancreatitis. The British Journal of Nutrition. 2009;**101**:787-793

[79] Zheng SY. Effects of early enteral nutrition on immune function of severe acute pancreatitis patients. World Journal of Gastroenterology. 2013;**19**:917-922

[80] Wereszczynska-Siemiatkowska U, Swidnicka-Siergiejko A, Siemiatkowski A, Dabrowski A. Early enteral nutrition is superior to delayed enteral nutrition for the prevention of infected necrosis and mortality in acute pancreatitis. Pancreas. 2013;**42**:640-646

[81] Li JY, Yu T, Chen GC, Yuan YH, Zhong W, Zhao LN, et al. Enteral nutrition within 48 hours of admission improves clinical outcomes of acute pancreatitis by reducing complications: A meta-analysis. PLoS One. 2013;**8**:e64926

[82] Qi D, Yu B, Huang J, Peng M. Meta-Analysis of Early Enteral Nutrition Provided Within 24 Hours of Admission on Clinical Outcomes in Acute Pancreatitis. JPEN J Parenter Enteral Nutr. 2018;**42**(7):1139-1147. DOI: 10.1002/jpen.1139

[83] Ramanathan M, Aadam AA. Nutrition management in acute pancreatitis. Nutrition in Clinical Practice. 2019;**34**(Suppl. 1):S7-S12

[84] Reddy BR. Enteral nutrition: Whom, why, when, what and where to feed? Nestle Nutrition Institute Workshop Series. 2015;**82**:53-59

[85] Windsor AC, Kanwar S, Li AG, Barnes E, Guthrie JA, Spark JI, et al. Compared with parenteral nutrition, enteral feeding attenuates the acute phase response and improves disease severity in acute pancreatitis. Gut. 1998;**42**:431-435

[86] Pupelis G, Selga G, Austrums E, Kaminski A. Jejunal feeding, even when instituted late, improves outcomes in patients with severe pancreatitis and peritonitis. Nutrition. 2001;**17**:91-94

[87] Makola D, Krenitsky J, Parrish C, Dunston E, Shaffer HA, Yeaton P, et al. Efficacy of enteral nutrition for the treatment of pancreatitis using standard enteral formula. The American Journal of Gastroenterology. 2006;**101**:2347-2355

[88] Cravo M, Camilo ME, Marques A. Early tube feeding in acute pancreatitis: A prospective study. Clinical Nutrition. 1989:A8-A14

[89] Tiegou LE, Gloro R, Pouzoulet J, et al. Semielemental formula or polymeric formula: Is there a better choice for enteral nutrition in acute pancreatitis? Randomized comparative study. JPEN Journal of Parenteral and Enteral Nutrition. 2006;**30**(1):1-5

[90] Spanier BW, Bruno MJ, Mathus-Vliegen EM. Enteral nutrition and acute pancreatitis: a review. Gastroenterol Res Pract. 2011;**2011**:857949. DOI: 10.1155/2011/857949. Epub 2010 Aug 3. PMID: 20811543; PMCID: PMC2929521

[91] He XL, Ma QJ, Lu JG, Chu YK, DuXL. Effect of total parenteral nutrition (TPN) with and without glutamine dipeptide supplementation on outcome in severe acute pancreatitis (SAP). Clinical Nutrition Supplements. 2004;**1**:43-47

[92] Mounzer R, Langmead CJ, Wu BU, et al. Comparison of existing clinical scoring systems to predict persistent organ failure in patients with acute pancreatitis. Gastroenterology. 2012;**142**:1476-1482

[93] Mier J, León EL, Castillo A, Robledo F, Blanco R. Early versus late necrosectomy in severe necrotizing pancreatitis. American Journal of Surgery. 1997;**173**:71-75

[94] McClave SA. Guidelines for the Provision and Assessment of Nutrition Support Therapy in the Adult Critically Ill Patient: Society of Critical Care Medicine (SCCM) and American Society for Parenteral and Enteral Nutrition (A.S.P.E.N.). JPEN Journal of Parenteral and Enteral Nutrition. 2016;**40**:159-211

[95] NICE-SUGAR Study Investigators. Intensive versus conventional glucose control in critically ill patients. The New England Journal of Medicine. 2009;**360**:1283-1297

[96] Khan R, Jehangir W, Regeti K, Yousif A. Hypertriglyceridemia-induced pancreatitis: Choice of treatment. Gastroenterology Research. 2015;**8**:234-236

[97] Mirtallo J, Canada T, Johnson D, Kumpf V, Petersen C, Sacks G, et al.

Safe practices for parenteral nutrition. JPEN Journal of Parenteral and Enteral Nutrition. 2004;**28**:S39-S70

[98] Setiawan VW, Pandol SJ, Porcel J, Wei PC, Wilkens LR, Le Marchand L, et al. Dietary factors reduce risk of acute pancreatitis in a large multiethnic cohort. Clinical Gastroenterology and Hepatology. 2017;**15**(2):257

[99] Al Samaraee A, McCallum IJ, Coyne PE, Seymour K. Nutritional strategies in severe acute pancreatitis: A systematic review of the evidence. The Surgeon. 2010;**8**(2):105-110

[100] Musil F, Zadak Z, Solichova D, Hyspler R, Kaska M, Sobotka L, et al. Dynamics of antioxidants in patients with acute pancreatitis and in patients operated for colorectal cancer: A clinical study. Nutrition. 2005;**21**:118-124

[101] Siriwardena AK, Mason JM, Balachandra S, Bagul A, Galloway S, Formela L, et al. Randomised, double blind, placebo controlled trial of intravenous antioxidant (n-acetylcysteine, selenium, vitamin C) therapy in severe acute pancreatitis. Gut. 2007;**56**:1439-1444

[102] Sateesh J, Bhardwaj P, Singh N, Saraya A. Effect of antioxidant therapy on hospital stay and complications in patients with early acute pancreatitis: A randomised controlled trial. Tropical Gastroenterology. 2009;**30**:201-206

[103] Du WD, Yuan ZR, Sun J, Tang JX, Cheng AQ, Shen DM, et al. Therapeutic efficacy of high-dose vitamin C on acute pancreatitis and its potential mechanisms. World Journal of Gastroenterology. 2003;**9**:2565-2569

[104] Bansal D, Bhalla A, Bhasin DK, Pandhi P, Sharma N, Rana S, et al. Safety and efficacy of vitamin-based antioxidant therapy in patients with severe acute pancreatitis: A randomized controlled trial. Saudi Journal of Gastroenterology. 2011;**17**:174-179

[105] Agah S, Akbari A, Sadeghi E, Morvaridzadeh M, Basharat Z, Palmowski A, et al. Resveratrol supplementation and acute pancreatitis: A comprehensive review. Biomedicine. 2021;**137**:111

[106] Hackert T, Werner J. Antioxidant therapy in acute pancreatitis: Experimental and clinical evidence. Antioxidants & Redox Signaling. 2011;**15**(10):2767-2777

[107] Özbeyli D, Gürler EB, Buzcu H, Çilingir-Kaya ÖT, Çam ME, Yüksel M. Astaxanthin alleviates oxidative damage in acute pancreatitis via direct antioxidant mechanisms. The Turkish Journal of Gastroenterology. 2020;**31**(10):706-712

[108] Jin TR. Curcumin and dietary polyphenol research: Beyond drug discovery. Acta Pharmacologica Sinica. 2018;**39**(5):779-786

[109] Huang S, Beevers CS. Pharmacological and clinical properties of curcumin. Botanics: Targets and Therapy. 2011;**1**:5-18

[110] Esatbeyoglu T, Huebbe P, Ernst IM, Chin D, Wagner AE, Rimbach G. Curcumin—From molecule to biological function. Angewandte Chemie (International Ed. in English). 2012;**51**(22):5308-5332

[111] Carmona-Ramirez I, Santamaria A, Tobon-Velasco JC, Orozco-Ibarra M, Gonzalez-Herrera IG, Pedraza-Chaverri J, et al. Curcumin restores Nrf2 levels and prevents quinolinic acid-induced neurotoxicity. The Journal of nutritional biochemistry. 2013;**24**(1):14-24

[112] Jagetia GC, Aggarwal BB. "Spicing up" of the immune system by curcumin. Journal of Clinical Immunology. 2007;**27**(1):19-35

[113] Lee W-H, Loo C-Y, Bebawy M, Luk F, Mason RS, Rohanizadeh R. Curcumin and its derivatives: Their application in neuropharmacology and neuroscience in the 21st century. Current Neuropharmacology. 2013;**11**:338-378

[114] Yu WG, Xu G, Ren GJ, Xu X, Yuan HQ, Qi XL, et al. Preventive action of curcumin in experimental acute pancreatitis in mouse. The Indian Journal of Medical research. 2011;**134**(5):717-724

[115] Durgaprasad S, Pai CG. A pilot study of the antioxidant effect of curcumin in tropical pancreatitis. The Indian journal of medical research. 2005;**122**(4):315-318

[116] Anchi P, Khurana A, Swain D, Samanthula G, Godugu C. Sustained-release curcumin microparticles for effective prophylactic treatment of exocrine dysfunction of pancreas: A preclinical study on cerulein-induced acute pancreatitis. Journal of Pharmaceutical Sciences. 2018;**107**(11):2869-2882

[117] Zhu Y et al. Gut microbiota dysbiosis worsens the severity of acute pancreatitis in patients and mice. Journal of Gastroenterology. 2019;**54**(4):347-358

[118] Brubaker L et al. Microbiome changes associated with acute and chronic pancreatitis: A systematic review. Pancreatology. 2021;**21**(1):1-14

[119] Zhang XM et al. Intestinal microbial community differs between acute pancreatitis patients and healthy volunteers. Biomedical and Environmental Sciences. 2018;**31**(1):81-86

[120] Rowland I et al. Gut microbiota functions: Metabolism of nutrients and other food components. European Journal of Nutrition. 2018;**57**(1):1-24

[121] Xu F, et al. The role of gut microbiota and genetic susceptibility in the pathogenesis of pancreatitis. Gut Liver; 2021

[122] Zhang YJ et al. Impacts of gut bacteria on human health and diseases. International Journal of Molecular Sciences. 2015;**16**(4):7493-7519

[123] Vancamelbeke M, Vermeire S. The intestinal barrier: A fundamental role in health and disease. Expert Review of Gastroenterology & Hepatology. 2017;**11**(9):821-834

[124] Zhu Y et al. Alteration of gut microbiota in acute pancreatitis and associated therapeutic strategies. Biomedicine & Pharmacotherapy. 2021;**141**:111850

[125] Lu WW et al. The role of gut microbiota in the pathogenesis and treatment of acute pancreatitis: A narrative review. Annals of Palliative Medicine. 2021;**10**(3):3445-3451

[126] Sawa H et al. Treatment outcome of selective digestive decontamination and enteral nutrition in patients with severe acute pancreatitis. Journal of Hepato-Biliary-Pancreatic Surgery. 2007;**14**(5):503-508

[127] Ahuja M et al. Orai1-mediated antimicrobial secretion from pancreatic acini shapes the gut microbiome and regulates gut innate immunity. Cell Metabolism. 2017;**25**(3):635-646

[128] Asrani V, Chang WK, Dong Z, Hardy G, Windsor JA, Petrov MS. Glutamine supplementation in acute pancreatitis: A meta-analysis

of randomized controlled trials. Pancreatology. 2013;**13**:468-474

[129] Yong L, Lu QP, Liu SH, Fan H. Efficacy of glutamine-enriched nutrition support for patients with severe acute pancreatitis: A meta-analysis. JPEN Journal of Parenteral and Enteral Nutrition. 2016;**40**:83-94

[130] Arutla M, Raghunath M, Deepika G, Jakkampudi A, Murthy HVV, Rao GV, et al. Efficacy of enteral glutamine supplementation in patients with severe and predicted severe acute pancreatitis—A randomized controlled trial. Indian Journal of Gastroenterology. 2019;**38**:338-347

[131] Liu X, Sun XF, Ge QX. The role of glutamine supplemented total parenteral nutrition (TPN) in severe acute pancreatitis. European Review for Medical and Pharmacological Sciences. 2016;**20**(19):4176-4180

[132] Monfared SSMS, Vahidi H, Abdolghaffari AH, Nikfar S, Abdollahi M. Antioxidant therapy in the management of acute, chronic and post-ERCP pancreatitis: A systematic review. World Journal of Gastroenterology. 2009;**15**:4481-4490

[133] Fuentes-Orozco C, Cervantes-Guevara G, Mucino-Hernandez I, LopezOrtega A, Ambriz-Gonzalez G, Gutierrez-de-la-Rosa JL, et al. L-alanyl-Lglutamine-supplemented parenteral nutrition decreases infectious morbidity rate in patients with severe acute pancreatitis. JPEN Journal of Parenteral and Enteral Nutrition. 2008;**32**:403-411

[134] Schwab JM, Serhan CN. Lipoxins and new lipid mediators in the resolution of inflammation. Current Opinion in Pharmacology. 2006;**6**(4):414-420

[135] Oskarsson V, Orsini N, Sadr-Azodi O, Wolk A. Fish consumption and risk of non-gallstone-related acute pancreatitis: A prospective cohort study. The American Journal of Clinical Nutrition. 2015;**101**:72-78

[136] Lasztity N, Hamvas J, Biro L, Nemeth E, Marosvolgyi T, Decsi T, et al. Effect of enterally administered n-3 polyunsaturated fatty acids in acute pancreatitis – a prospective randomized clinical trial. Clinical Nutrition. 2005;**24**:198-205

[137] Wang X, Li W, Li N, Li J. Omega-3 fatty acids-supplemented parenteral nutrition decreases hyperinflammatory response and attenuates systemic disease sequelae in severe acute pancreatitis: A randomized and controlled study. JPEN Journal of Parenteral and Enteral Nutrition. 2008;**32**:236-241

[138] Xiong J, Zhu S, Zhou Y, Wu H, Wang C. Regulation of omega-3 fish oil emulsion on the SIRS during the initial stage of severe acute pancreatitis. J Huazhong Univ Sci Technolog Med Sci. 2009;**29**(1):35-38. DOI: 10.1007/s11596-009-0107-3